The Hospice Heart
A journey I didn't have a map for
❖
By Gabrielle Elise Jimenez

"My memories say hello... they ask about you all the time"

Make more memories...

Every day I feel such gratitude for the work I do and the people I do it with and for; all of you are my teachers. I hope to learn something new every day; by no means do I think I know it all. We can never know it all. I've been taught well and generously by some of the best and I hold those lessons very close to my heart.

I know how blessed I am.

I am thankful to all of the patients I have been present for,

and to their families who have trusted them in my care.

To my family and friends, who support and encourage me every day, I say thank you. I know how hard it is to be around me sometimes. I know I make you cry when I share my stories...but hopefully I also make you feel. I love you so much xo

Working in hospice I have learned that life is fragile, beautiful, difficult and kind...but can sometimes be mean. I have learned that love is a beautiful thing but is always being tested. I have learned that we are all so much stronger than we give ourselves credit. I have learned that faith, for some and even for those who never practice, truly can bring comfort, safety and peace. I have learned that a Popsicle is a gift, that a cool cloth on a warm forehead is magical, and that sitting by the bedside of someone who is struggling so that if/when they open their eyes and see you.... know they are not alone... is kind. And I have learned, that holding a hand says so much more than words.

Most of all though... I have learned that life is amazing and beautiful and no one knows how much of it will be ours so we need to treasure each moment, be kinder to one another, let the little stuff go, stop being mean and hurtful and realize that words cannot be taken back so be very mindful of what you say. And most of all... appreciate all you have.

In my first book Soft Landing, I wanted to share the journey I took to becoming a nurse. I think part of me wanted to inspire others not to give up on a goal simply because of a few obstacles, but I also think it was important to share how and why my passion is so deep relative to hospice care and the work I do. Writing that book was therapy for me; I evolved so much during that period between starting nursing school and working with patients at the end of their life. It felt really good to be able to write it down and share it.

Being a hospice nurse fills my soul on so many levels; I feel blessed and honored to do the work I do but also to be able to meet so many incredible people. Every day I am exposed to the fragility of life, the power of human kindness and compassion and strength and resilience that blows my mind. All of these things inspire me to continue to do what I do.

In Soft Landing I share that I was laid off from a job I thought I would be doing the rest of my life, and ended up caring for a friend who was dying, which is what started this path I am on today. But I have come to realize that I was already on the path at a very young age and had absolutely no idea. How funny it is to think you are where you are supposed to be only to end up somewhere completely different and then come to the realization that this is where you were meant to be all along. Does that make sense? I needed to go through all of that to get here, and while it wasn't easy, it was surely worth it.

My Childhood

As a young girl, I would play with Troll dolls instead of Barbie's. I was more of an outside kid and I liked to play in the dirt. I would build these cave homes in the hillside for my Trolls and spend hours and hours creating adventures for them. The most common was playing nurse. One of my Trolls was always the nurse and she had a special cave that the other Trolls would come to for help when they were injured or sick. I also played with plastic horses, so usually one of my Trolls would fall off or get kicked by the horses and would need to be bandaged up by the nurse (me).

When I was a teenager, my father shared property in Comptche; which was a very small town. It was about three miles to the nearest road, seven miles to the nearest town (which consisted of a grocery store, a gas pump and a mail stop) and twenty-five miles to Mendocino. We did not have electricity, our bathroom was an outhouse and our light was a kerosene lamp. I lived out in the middle of nowhere and nature was my playground. There were all kinds of creek beds and cool wooded forests that welcomed my imagination on a daily basis. I built a mini hospital in one of the creek beds and my brothers and sisters were my patients; sometimes they would have (pretend) broken bones, always cuts and bruises and a few times I was called in for surgery and had to remove a splinter or two. I was a nurse, I was their nurse, and I loved it.

As I became an adult and started living on my own, I was the go-to person when someone had a scrape or a burn; my drawers always had band aids, gauze, medical tape and Neosporin, I could have been a spokesperson for Neosporin, it served so many purposes.

As a young person, I always reacted sensitively to someone else who was hurting, whether it was emotionally or physically. I was drawn very early on to provide compassionate care.

My First Death

When I was about eight years old, a young man on his motorcycle, came around the corner near my house. I was in my bedroom and I can remember very clearly hearing the motorcycle roaring closely and then I heard the crash, and then I heard silence. He had come around the corner and hit the tree so hard he went one way and the bike went another. I ran out of my house and right up to him, I wasn't afraid and while it didn't even occur to me then, I must have had some instinct because I immediately fell to my knees, took the sweatshirt from around my waste and tied it around his leg to catch all the blood. There was so much blood.

I placed his head in my lap and I remember slowly smoothing out his hair and telling him that help was on the way. I am not even sure how I knew that, or whether or not help was actually on the way but it seemed at the time, the right thing to say. I remember hearing sirens shortly after and soon paramedics were at the site. A neighbor grabbed me and pulled me away.

I watched as they all moved around him quickly opening packages of things, and paper flying around and sounds of beeping and activity that felt chaotic. I just stood there and watched. I don't recall being scared; in fact I don't think I really felt anything at all, except for wondering where his parents were... I kept thinking his parents really should be there. Which is ironic, because my parents were not there, I was not being supported by family. I was alone, on the side of the street near my home, in the arms of a neighbor.

All of a sudden there was silence, and the team of paramedics that were working on him started to stand up and back away. I watched as they got him up on a gurney, covering him completely and putting him in the ambulance. The police that had arrived during all of this, started to clean up the trash and debris left on the ground. I watched as it took two people to pick up the mangled motorcycle and move it to the side of the road. And then I watched as one of them picked up my ragged yellow sweatshirt that was soaked through with blood and toss it in the trash. Of course I didn't want it, but no one even asked if I did.

No one really seemed to know that I was still there, or that this might have effected me somehow, or that I was there when he first crashed and held his head in my lap. I imagine now, that he must have died that day, quite possibly while in my lap. I don't remember anything after that day, any stories that were told, or questions being asked. I don't remember my family discussing it. I do remember always looking at that tree with a very lengthy gaze each time I passed it by. And now, looking back, I remember how much sense it made to comfort him.

I was such a brave and fearless little hippie girl back then, filled with so much empathy. I had no idea what death meant, or how permanent it was, but I was always the first one to nurse a bird with a broken wing, getting squished insects to safety and always feeling bad for anyone with cuts or bruises, or worse, broken bones. But death… I did not have much experience with. That young man, who died after crashing his motorcycle near my house, was my first death and my initial reaction was to run to his side and provide comfort, and relieve him of fear. I truly believe that was the first moment my heart started making itself open to hospice.

My Father

Growing up, I didn't have a very emotional relationship with my father. As a child I felt abandoned and abused, but as an adult who had a lot of therapy I realize now that he did the best he could. I worked hard to get there. I spent a lot of my youth trying to get his attention, to get him to acknowledge my good parts. I always felt like I wasn't good enough, that I was a failure and I would never amount to anything worthwhile. This is a very heavy weight to carry for someone so young. I understand now, that much of my struggle, was self-inflicted but at that age my whole world seemed like one disappointment after another and I felt those feelings in a very big way. It dictated how I treated myself and what I allowed in my life. If only we could call a do over!

My dad was a very talented cabinet-maker and I would spend hours and hours sitting in his woodshop, inhaling the wonderful aroma of saw dust as he worked and I did homework or drew. I never told him this, but when we would go to install cabinets, redwood doors with stained glassed windows, and even church pews, I would watch in awe as he created so much beauty. I would slowly run my fingers over the soft wood, stare out the stained glass, and even kneel gently on the pew and think to myself "my dad did this". But I never told him that. I wish I had.

When I was in my twenties, my dad was diagnosed with Guillain Barre Syndrome; an illness that at the time was not something the doctors knew a lot about. Not being medically savvy, I saw it as an illness that deadened his nerve endings, curling his fingers and toes making it difficult for him to do things like tying his shoes, or pulling up a zipper. I saw a strong man become weak and dependent on others for self-care, but at the time I had no understanding or comprehension about death so it was never a thought that entered my brain.

When he got sick I tried to be there for him the best that I could. I would drive him to appointments and run errands for him. In retrospect, I could have done more. His illness progressed rapidly, he was in and out of hospitals and he went from being flat on his back in a hospital bed, to using his walking sticks and driving. So I was confused about his prognosis and again, not aware that he could die or even what that might look like or mean. This went on for several years.

One thanksgiving he called to ask if he could come have dinner with my kids and I. At that time I was hosting a dinner for all of my friends who had nowhere to go. I went and picked him up and brought him to my home. Before eating dinner, I had everyone say something they were thankful for. When it came time for my dad to speak, he looked at me and said, "I am thankful for my daughter. I am so proud of her and how hard she works. She is a wonderful mother and a wonderful daughter". I cried, of course. I had waited so many years to hear these words. I am pretty sure this was the very best day of my life as his daughter.

I drove him home the next morning. He asked me to stay but I had plans with friends and needed to go. He asked if I would just stay for lunch, but I declined. All the way back home I felt bad, and I felt guilty. I called him that night to apologize for leaving so quickly, offering to come by the next day for lunch. I did not hear back from him. I left another message, offering to bring lunch to him, to run any errands he needed. No response. The next day I received a call from his sister asking me to come to the hospital, as he was taken the night before because he had gotten very sick. I rushed to the hospital. He was in a hospital bed dying. At one point, I remember everyone had stepped out of the room and I sat on a bench about ten feet away just watching him breathe. His breathing was slow, not labored and almost peaceful. And then as I sat there I felt a shift of the energy in the room, I knew he was taking his last breaths. I didn't move from the bench, I didn't go to his bedside; I didn't hold his hand or let him know I was there. I just sat there and stared, almost numb. I felt his spirit leave his body. I felt my dad leave this life. And he died.

I knew I had missed all the right chances to have last words, to say goodbye, to let things go. I know that I held on to my anger so tightly, nothing else could have come through. I regret this every single day. This has haunted me most of my life. Perhaps it has also inspired me in that the one thing I always encourage anyone sitting at the bedside to do, is to say goodbye, but also to say "thank you", "I'm sorry", or even "I forgive you". Or better yet, don't wait for the bedside to say those things. Say them while they can be heard and appreciated, while they can make a difference in the relationship, and perhaps even change the future you could have together, however long or short it may be.

After my dad passed away, we went to clean out his room. I noticed the message light blinking on his answering machine, so I pushed "play". I heard the messages I left, the messages he never heard. At that moment I realized that he never knew I called, or that I tried to see him or that I felt really bad for not staying the day before. I have stored so much regret inside and every time I see someone at the bedside feeling guilt for not doing or saying something sooner, I am reminded.

Guilt is a painful thing. I have tried to let it go, and for the most part I have, but I feel compelled now to do what I can to make sure that no one else feels this way. We do this to ourselves, we beat ourselves up over things we should have or could have done. This is not a healthy practice. There is no written "right" or "wrong" way to be there for someone at death. The truth is that everyone is different; their needs and wants are different.

Sure I could have done things differently for him, but that was a long time ago and I didn't know then what I know now. I had to learn and grow and I truly believe that this journey I have been on has helped me to see him and the gifts he brought into my life, to truly appreciate the man he was and while I didn't see it then, I see our similarities and I like them. Maybe his gift to me was the spark that started to light up inside me to eventually get me where I am today. Thank you Dad.

My Mother

My mother died before my father. She was diagnosed with lung cancer and yes, she was a very heavy smoker. I remember cleaning up over-flowing ashtrays on her bedside table, and sometimes, removing a cigarette from her fingers when she fell asleep smoking in bed. Her cancer spread quickly and she was given one year to live. I was twenty-five years old and had no idea what this meant, but having two parents nearing the end of their life was a lot for someone so young, At this same time I was a single mother raising a five year old. I lived about four hours away from my mother so I didn't see her very often and much like my relationship with my dad, we were not close. Something else I regret. It felt as though she went from diagnosis to death in a matter of seconds, but true to her "year to live" time frame, she died almost exactly one year from being told that.

When my mother passed away she wanted to be cremated, something else I knew absolutely nothing about. At the time I was working for a Corian company and decided to design and create a Corian urn for her. It was actually very pretty once finished and when I took it to the funeral home, they loved it and asked if I would make them some. That was the start of a business that took off running. I called my company RuCor (Ruth, my mom's name, plus Corian), I got a patent for my design and I sold Corian urns from Monterey to Mendocino. I visited every mortuary, crematorium, funeral home and cemetery I could find. I went to conferences and tradeshows and learned a lot about burial, but nothing about death. I met the nicest people and was pleasantly surprised to see that Morticians and Funeral Directors were not morbid or dark as I had imagined and in fact were gentle and kind and almost funny at times, always having a one-liner along the lines of "people are just dying to come here".

I really enjoyed selling urns, but the business got too big for me and I made the decision to sell it and the Patent at a ridiculously low amount. I wish I knew then what I know now; I would have kept the business, asked for guidance on how to run a big business and perhaps I would be quite wealthy now. But alas… things did not turn out that way.

They Used To Call Me "Cemetery Girl"

Seriously. It's true. Even as a really young kid, I was fascinated and drawn to cemeteries. As a young kid, leaving the house and not coming back until dark wasn't such a big deal, and I would walk and walk for what seemed like hours. I liked to explore. I had two favorite places, the dump and the cemetery. Don't get grossed out… the dump was cool; people threw away the most wonderful treasures, and it allowed my imagination to go full speed ahead. I used to look for suitcases in hopes a bank robber was running from the cops and threw it in the dump planning to come back and get it. But I would find it and I would come home with so much money and oh… the things we could have. But that is a whole other story.

The cemetery was my safe place, I was never afraid going there. I would walk through it, looking at all the headstones creating stories about each person buried there and the life they had before they died. I would wonder about their families and how they might be doing. At each visit, I would pick my "favorite" headstone and plop down next to it; I would unwrap my peanut butter and jelly sandwich and I would have a picnic. I always brought bubbles and after my lunch, I would sit and blow bubbles until I ran out.

This is where I got the nickname; the groundskeepers gave it to me… as I would walk by them they would say "hi cemetery girl" and laugh. I think they were being mean, but it didn't faze me. This was after I had been going for quite some time; initially they told me I shouldn't be there and once the taller guy told me that sometimes bodies come out of the dirt and grab little girls… I am not sure why that didn't scare me off.

To this day, I find such peace at a cemetery and will often pull over when I see one and walk the grounds for a bit, just thinking about all the lives that were put to rest there.

I didn't know it then, but I think all of that started me on this journey of working as a hospice nurse. It's funny how things work out the way they do, how you can suddenly be at this place in your life and have no idea how the hell you got there and yet… you realize you do know… it just took a little while to see all the roads that actually took me here.

I believe that the lessons I learned from having two terminally ill parents die within months of one another were not clear earlier on because I wasn't ready yet to see them. Perhaps I chose not to, I will never know. But from that moment to this one, there has been a lot of growth for me and I realize that while I am in the right place for me, I am a continuous work in progress. I am on a journey I don't have a map for but I am finding my way.

I started a blog because I felt I had so much to say about the care of someone at the end of life. Hospice nursing is only minimally taught in schools and while there are websites and podcasts and books on gentle care, I feel that often times it's the little simple things that anyone can do for someone when they are dying. You don't need a license to do mouth care, or provide tactile stimuli or verbal comfort. The second half of this book contains my first blog postings. I cover everything from bedside care, to patient stories, and my own personal thoughts about death and life and lessons I have learned along the way.

For me, my most powerful lesson has been learning how to be fully present for someone else, and understanding what that really means. We are not taught this, we experience this and the full understanding of it all continues to evolve within me.

What Does It Mean To Be Present?

Being present is not something that just magically happens because someone suggests you do it, and in my opinion, it is not something we are born with and just know. I am speaking from my perspective only; from what I have seen, what I have experienced and what I have learned. It takes practice, commitment and intention. I understand that what worked for me, might not work for someone else and you might read my words and roll your eyes or think to yourself, "I can't do this" but what if you can? Imagine the difference you can make for someone else when you truly learn the art of being present.

Have you ever had a conversation with someone and wondered what they said after it was over, or read a book you got fifty pages in before realizing you had no idea what it was about? It is because you checked out, you thought about something else, got distracted, and perhaps even lost interest. For me, being present is learning how to stay focused on what it is I am doing at that time. So I started there. I became aware of when I would drift off and I learned how to bring myself back. I paid more attention to conversations, listening to what was being said, and truly hearing the words being spoken.

Someone told me once to get grounded, which I had to Google. It meant so many different things I had a hard time relating it to being present so I found myself a little confused. And then someone else said, "no silly, feel the ground" and proceeded to teach me how to meditate and connect with the earth, to feel the power beneath my feet, and allow it to help me find balance and peace. This took work, but when I finally felt "it", it was incredible.

In an effort to continue to learn ways that I can be fully present, I started to attend Healing Touch classes, which is an energy-based approach to health and healing, it helped me to really connect with the energy of another. I have read that some say Hospice and Healing Touch is a "match made in heaven" and I have to agree. I was first introduced to Healing Touch when our volunteers would come and without words or touch, were able to calm an agitated patient who was struggling in their last hours of life. They would bring a sense of peace and comfort that medication was not capable of doing. I would sit back quietly in awe of their ability to connect so deeply to someone else, simply by being present. And while it is a true benefit to our patients, it also brought comfort to those at the bedside. Healing Touch works on anyone, whether they are near death or not.

I wanted to have my own personal "rituals" that would help me to achieve being present before seeing my patients, so I started by taking a few deep breaths before entering a patient's room, shaking off whatever might be weighing on me, heavy or otherwise. Making sure that when I walk into someone else's space, I am 100% there and completely present. Once I started being completely present, I realized that I wasn't just listening, I was hearing and I wasn't just seeing, I was feeling, and most importantly, I made this about them, and not me.

Another thing I have found to be really helpful, at least for me, is reflection. I start each day setting nine intentions for my day, whether it is to be more patient, or less judgmental, or to not yell at horrible drivers. And at the end of the day, I reflect. I think about the day, the people I saw and the things I did, but most importantly, the patients I cared for and the deaths I might have attended. I reflect on how I felt at whatever experience might have transpired and I work through it. I have found that when I do that, I do not carry it into the next day or with the people and paths I might come across. It reduces my distractions and allows me to be more focused.

For me, being present in my work, means being totally committed to someone else, at their time of need, honoring them with the very best care and compassion to allow for a death that can truly be called peaceful, beautiful and good. Being present means sitting quietly at the bedside, saying absolutely nothing, except for "I am right here" when they flinch in pain, or moan or cry out for someone to acknowledge they are not alone. Being present means being fully aware of what is going on around me, it means not projecting my energy onto someone else, and it means not allowing outside forces to effect the peacefulness I find or thrive for, within.

Being present for me outside of work, means to be a better listener, and to pick up on that moment when my friend or family member is asking for my help. It means to learn when I've pushed myself too far or too hard and did not set boundaries, which can only bring on stress or anxiety. It means listening to my body, and taking care of me, something I am constantly working on. And most of all, it means to remember that everything is not about me. I admit it; I am a constant work in progress.

I have many "rituals" that work for me; I take a lot of deep breaths, I plant my feet firmly on the ground, I wiggle my toes and my fingers and I shake off anything that might be distracting and I embrace the moment completely. That is what being present means to me. To be trusted at the bedside of someone nearing the end of their life is an honor and I believe that in order to respect that gift, it is our responsibility to be fully and completely present for them. I understand now what that means.

I want to share with you something that has really resonated with me. It is a book called Vigil, The Poetry of Presence, by Pamela Heinrich MacPherson. She is a hospice volunteer who has done beautiful work, which her words reflect so wonderfully. www.vigilpoetry.com

From her poem "Winding Down"

> Time. It takes time.
> An open-hearted, focused presence
> Is what we can bring.
> A compassionate and loving gift
> In these last days, hours and moments.
> It is all.
> It is sacred.
> It is enough…

Is It Our Experience Or Theirs?

One of our biggest mistakes is projecting how we feel or what we need onto someone else who doesn't have a voice. The purpose of this book is to help others find ways to provide comfort, care and support to someone as they are nearing the last days of their life.

Little things like how hot or cold you might feel, does not necessarily reflect how someone else feels, especially someone lying in a bed at the end of their life. I understand this might not be clinically correct and there are many people that might disagree, but I have found that checking hands and feet does not adequately determine whether someone is hot or cold internally. Sometimes, a cool extremity is based on loss of oxygen and most commonly a sign of near death. It is a good way to gage how close a person might be. But sometimes they just have cold hands and feet. I have noticed that if I touch the arms or legs of someone and they are warm, it indicates to me they might be more comfortable with a sheet over them, as opposed to five blankets.

It seems almost automatic to place blankets on someone who isn't feeling well; we think it provides them comfort and most of the time it does, but what if it makes them more uncomfortable? If they can verbalize their needs, ask them. Always ask them. The most important thing you can do for someone who is going through this process is to allow him or her to have a choice. And choosing between a thick layer of blankets or a cool soft sheet is a choice. If they cannot verbalize, feel their skin, and decide then what you think they might need.

I was sitting with a patient once, who was actively dying. I sat with him for hours. He was a very religious person; his faith was strong and provided him comfort. Where I do have my own spiritual connection and am constantly growing in that area, until I became a hospice nurse did I truly understand the depths of people's faith, beliefs and support they receive from their prayers and prayer communities.

My patient was verbally non-responsive. He could not tell me whether he wanted music or silence or to be touched or left alone. So I sat there.... holding his hand and staying quiet, yet completely present in his experience. I saw his prayer book on the table next to his bed; I picked it up and started to read it to him. I read every single page. I feel like I brought him comfort but what surprised me most, was the comfort it brought me.

This experience, and most of my bedside moments with patients at the end of their lives, reminds me that it's not about us. It is very easy to get incredibly wrapped up in whatever you feel, think, or need and it is very easy to project that onto others. It takes practice learning to let that go... learning to allow other people to have their own experiences, choices, and life practices without feeling compelled to "correct" or redirect them.

He passed incredibly peacefully and I find comfort knowing I contributed to that. I also found comfort in reading to him prayers that are not of a faith I follow but a faith he follows and at that moment when it mattered most... it was absolutely 100% about him.

Some Days Can Be Really Difficult In This Line Of Work

When I walked in her room, she was alone. She was struggling for breath, and she was dying. There were two beds in her room, one of which I assumed was her son's as I heard he was there visiting with her. Staff at the facility told me he had gone for a walk. I administered some Morphine and Lorazepam, two medications that play nicely together, especially at the end of life. They were mildly effective; her breathing was calmed but she was definitely transitioning. I left her there, thinking I wished she wasn't alone. I spoke to the floor nurse at her facility and asked them to please check in on her, and to call us for any changes in her condition. And for the next two hours as I visited with other patients, I thought about her and I struggled with the thought of her being alone.

But then I got a call asking me to go back, to provide continuous care at her bedside because she was actively dying. I was so happy I could go back to her, to help relieve her struggle and to comfort her until she passed.

When I arrived, I was greeted by five of her six sons, and a few other extended family members. And her husband of sixty-one years was at her bedside holding her hand. He was tearful and fully present half of the time and the other half his dementia took hold and he was confused and couldn't quite comprehend what was happening, which was painful to watch for everyone in the room.

Her breathing was labored and she fought her death every second I was there. It took me five hours but I was finally able to manage her symptoms with medication and I educated the family on how to provide tactile stimuli, love, kindness and care to work in tandem with the medication. They did a beautiful job.

I watched as her sons struggled to find the right words to say to her but also to one another. I watched as they each handled this their own way, and noticed how fragile they were. I watched, as grown men became small boys and how much they loved their mom and didn't have the strength to say goodbye. So I gathered them all together and I encouraged them to remember. To remember their lives growing up and the wonderful times they had with her. I encouraged them to go back in her room and go to that place within where memories are stored, to share those things with her and tell her thank you for the wonderful life she gave them. And they did. And it was beautiful. I encouraged them to each give her a goodbye message as well, to let her know that they would be okay and would take care of one another and mostly, that they would take care of their dad. One at a time they gave her a personal message.

Just before she took her last breaths, I called them all back in. They gathered around the bed, very tearful and very connected, each touching the other, holding hands, arms wrapped around shoulders and hugging. Her husband, their father, was at her bedside holding her hand and crying. They asked what they should do, and because of her strong spiritual beliefs, I encouraged prayer and they decided to say the Hale Mary prayers. She took her last breath as they finished it the fifth time. It was beautiful, it was peaceful and it was without distress or struggle. And they cried, and cried, and cried.

I was standing in the back of the room, holding back my own tears, and I slowly made my way to her bedside to confirm that she had passed, even though I already knew. I put my stethoscope to my ear and the other end to her heart and I listened to silence. I looked up at each of them confirming what they too already knew. And then I looked at her husband. He was staring at me with dime-sized tears in his eyes. And then it hit him; he realized his wife just died. He was clear and confused at the same time and he needed someone to take it out on. He started to yell at me "you liar" and he repeated it several times, each one louder than the one before.

My heart ached, and I cried and I kept saying, "I am so sorry" because I didn't know what else to say. I stood there and let him yell at me because I knew he needed to let it out but each word felt like stabs at my chest. One of her son's took my hand and walked me out of the room and hugged me for what seemed like forever. He kept apologizing for his father and thanking me for being there. He told me not to take his fathers words personally. He said words to me that I say to everyone else "this isn't about you" and it resonated deep.

I walked into the other room and I did my paperwork, I called the funeral home, I updated everyone that needed to know and I gathered my things. I went to say goodbye to the family. Their father's wheelchair had its back to me so I was hoping to slip out swiftly so he didn't notice. But the family had other plans, the sons had other plans and they each took turns giving me tight, loving hugs; each thanking me for being there. Her granddaughter came up to me and hugged me, her eyes filled with tears and she too apologized for her grandpa. I explained that it wasn't needed, that I understood, but I realized as she said it, maybe I did need it, so I thanked her for her words. And then he turned his wheelchair around to see what all the fuss was about. We connected eyes. I was afraid for a moment that he would yell again. But he looked at me and he apologized, and then he said, "I have loved her my whole life. I am going to miss her so much". And he took my hand and asked me to sit. So I curled up on the floor next to his wheel chair and we both cried.

As I left them that day and walked down the hallway to the elevator, I started to cry. And then, which came as quite a surprise to me, I started to say the Hale Mary prayer, something, of which I never quite understood until that day. And I felt peace. And I felt okay with everything that took place that day. I knew I did good work for my patient, for the family and for her husband.

I Am Exactly Where I Am Supposed To Be

I had the most powerful dream one morning. I had slept a full night, woken up at six AM by the sprinklers and the sun shining through my window, and I liked it. I thought how lucky I am that I have the ability to hear and to see and to feel all the things that are happening around me. And as it was only six AM, and I was off that day and didn't have to get up early, I decided to nap a little longer, sink deeper under my cozy comforter and see where the sleep would take me.

My dream, as I can tell by the time it was when I woke up, was probably about thirty minutes. I was outside in a field, with really high grasses, and lots of trees and it was peaceful and it felt good. I felt like I was exactly where I was supposed to be. It was intentional. I didn't see it coming up but I wasn't surprised by it being there. It was this beautiful brown horse with a black mane flowing wildly with the wind, his thick hairs hitting me gently in the face. He had a patch of white on his forehead and the most beautiful, most peaceful, and most inviting eyes that made me feel safe. He kept nudging me, trying to get my attention. I pet his face and kissed his nose. He kept nudging me, getting as close as he possibly could to me. I kept asking him what he wanted, as though I knew he was trying to tell me something. And then I heard "everything is going to be exactly how it is supposed to be. You are where you are supposed to be. You are doing what you are meant to do". In my dream I could hear those words so clearly.

I didn't feel him leave, I didn't see him walk away, but I was suddenly alone, back in this grassy field filled with trees. But I didn't feel alone. I felt safe. Most of all I felt excited because I knew... I was exactly where I was supposed to be.

And then I woke up. And for the first time in my entire life, everything felt like it has fallen perfectly in place. Perhaps he was right... I am exactly where I am supposed to be. Life has a funny way of letting you know that while there might be obstacles or things are not exactly how you intended or even hoped they would be, they are exactly what they are meant to be and I realize that now with my career path.

The Last Goodbye

I was sitting with a wife, two daughters and a son of a patient who was dying. It is at this time that I have the conversation about what to say to someone before they die. I have this conversation often, and while the information I give is usually the same, the reactions and the responses from families vary. "Your husband needs to know that you will be okay", I said. I have said this more times than I can count. It made sense to me. But this time was different; his wife said to me "but I am not going to be okay". And at that moment, I came to the realization that I need to think about what I say, and what is truly appropriate for each situation. How the heck do I know what he needs from her, his wife of sixty years, and who am I to say she will be okay. Of course she will not be okay. I would not be okay. I looked at her and I looked into her eyes and I could see how scared she was, how sad she was and I knew, she doesn't want to do this, she does not want to know how to say goodbye to her husband, whom she still loves very much and more than anything, wants more time with.

We spent some time talking about him, the kind of man he has been all of their lives and what they think he would want. I asked if it would be more appropriate to let him know they will take care of their mother. They agreed that was exactly what he needed reassurance for; he would want to know that after he was gone, they would all make sure she was taken care of. We talked about one of the things people always seem to say; "he will be in a better place" and how on many levels, that is just absurd. A better place, at least in their eyes, was there, with them and him no longer ill or in pain. I gave great thought to that as well.

After I left them that day, I really thought about the last goodbye, the last words, and things I would want to know and hear. It reminded me of a class I took with Shaman Linda Fitch; it was about crossing over and we did a "Sacred Deathbed" exercise. She asked if I would like to volunteer for the first one, and then everyone would pair up and do it in groups. I had no idea what was going to happen, but who says "no" to the Shaman, right? I waited downstairs while the class of nine people prepared for what ended up being my death.

When I walked into the room, I was no longer with my classmates, instead they were all representing my children, my friends and someone from my past who would be the one to take my hand as I crossed over. This exercise was more powerful than I ever could have imagined and it has stayed very present within me ever since. At my deathbed, my children said goodbye. They cried as they asked me not to leave, and I could feel their pain as they said goodbye to me. Saying goodbye to them was so permanent, I think that is the best word to describe it, because that kind of goodbye, the one at the deathbed, is forever. I died that day and my soul rose above the room and watched as the people I love grieved, as they read the Eulogy I wrote, and as they said their final goodbye to me.

Several things came out of that exercise for me; most importantly is that I am not ready to go quite yet and that my love for my children, my family and my friends is a deep, beautiful love and I am grateful. I also realized that while I wish I could have done some things differently in my lifetime, I do not have regrets, I do not have a need for a "do-over" and I don't feel there are words I could have, or should have said to someone. I felt very at peace with my life and the path I was on. I realized that at my deathbed, there would be no need for apologies or forgiveness and that gave me a sense of relief.

This got me thinking about how so many times, humans wait for the beside to say the things they could have or should have said earlier. What if we didn't? What if we didn't hold grudges, what if we let things go, what if we said the kind words, the reassuring words, and the supportive and loving words so much when we felt them, that at the deathbed… you already knew. And the only thing that really needs to be said is "I will miss you".

I was with another family just before their mother/wife took her last breaths. They asked me what they should say. I told them to tell her thank you for the wonderful gifts she gave them during their time together, and let her know how much she will be missed. I walked out of the room to give them time to say goodbye and I heard their lovely words. The last things she heard, besides the beautiful music playing in the background, was "thank you" and "we will miss you".

Don't wait for the bedside to say the things… don't hold grudges, or hang onto anger. Instead, embrace your life right now, and all the people you have in it. Make moments and memories and love fiercely.

The next pages of my book are all of my blogs from when I first started it. Writing the blog was very cathartic for me, and very healing. Every day I spend with a patient and their friends or family, I take something away with me. Sometimes it is the comfort knowing I was helpful, sometimes the reminder of why I do this work, but most times it's lessons and reminders of how to live a full life, a kind life, a life filled with compassion.

My wish for each of you, after reading this book, is that you too have a take away; that you feel good inside, and your heart feels touched. Perhaps I can inspire you to do this work, or maybe just help you feel more confident in the care you are providing a loved one. You are a wonderful human being, you have a heart so full and there is kindness within, I know this to be true. Share it with others, even in the smallest of ways. Raise your head up when walking down the street and smile at the person heading your way, hold a door open, wait your turn, be patient, let someone cut in front of the line, and don't get mad if they do. Take deep breaths often, whatever will be, will be… accept that. Be kind to yourself and be kind to others, and do great work in this wonderful crazy world, and make a positive difference!!

Joy

Joy is

the gift

we give ourselves

through

gratefulness.

By Charles M. Fontenot, his book "In Search Of My Soul"

My blog: The Hospice Heart

www.thehospiceheart.net

Every Sunday I add a new blog, and I usually wait until the very last minute to decide what I am going to write about. So many things inspire me; my visits with patients and their families, conversations I have with coworkers and the lessons that each human I am lucky to cross paths with, teaches me.

The blogs I am sharing with you here, were the first that I wrote. I invite you to visit my blog every week, and see what has transpired since I published this book. I hope to continue to learn and grow, and have many more amazing experiences that I will share with all of you.

You will find that I repeat myself, and sometimes there is a frequent common thread; I just think that sometimes things need to be said more than once.

Hospice Is Not A Diagnosis; It Is A Plan Of Care For The Diagnosis

What is hospice? I get asked this question a lot. I have also heard the many misconceptions about what hospice is, and I have seen fear, a lot of fear. To many people, hospice is a death sentence and it is dark and scary and means there is no turning back... you are going to die. And this is true, because when given the hospice order, it means you have received a terminal diagnosis with the assumption you have 6 months or less to live. Could that change? Yes. I have seen people thrive and get off of hospice. I love that, I hope for that. Unfortunately, it doesn't happen often. But hospice isn't the diagnosis, it isn't the death sentence; hospice is a plan of care. It is the gathering of a team that together find a way to support the patient and the family during what will be the hardest time of their life.

When I start seeing a patient, they are already on hospice; they are already aware of their diagnosis, their prognosis, and the inevitable way things will turn out. I wish so badly that I could change the outcome; I think all of us working in this field feel the same way. But we can't, and we are realistic about that. What we can do, however, is make sure that you always feel supported, that you are relieved of pain and distress, that you are provided the supplies, the medications, the education and support you and your loved ones need to work through this process.

Most of you have heard the names Frank Ostaseski, BJ Miller, Jessica Zitter, Barbara Karnes, Katy Butler, and my personal favorite, Gary Pasternak. These are all people I have listened to, read their books and followed as they shared their lessons about the end of life. There are so many more I could name and all of them have found a way to raise the dark cloud off "hospice", just enough for me to realize that death, while painful, scary and terrifying, can actually be beautiful.

They are the ones who have taught me about what bedside manner truly means, how compassion plays such a key role at the end of life and how as humans we need to practice more kindness and learn the true meaning of being present. These people are not angels they are human beings who give completely to other human beings going through a difficult experience. I respect and admire them and I am grateful to them for showing me the way.

I certainly can't speak for anyone else that works in this field, but for myself I can say that there is no end to what I can learn and how I can grow and how excited that makes me feel. I want to learn more, I want to continue to grow and to be able to not only provide a kinder experience for my patient's and their families, but to also share what I am given to others just starting out. We are a community of people who give our hearts freely and without need for anything in return, except perhaps the knowledge that we might have made a difference in a difficult experience and truly provided the soft landing every human being deserves to have.

We are all going to die, and there is no rhyme or reason how one is chosen over another or how short or long our time will be. But the one thing we can choose is how we are treated and cared for when that time comes. I can assure you that if you are given a terminal diagnosis and you go on hospice, there will be a team that will work collaboratively to ensure the care you and your loved ones receive is compassionate and kind.

It's Not About You

The first thing you have to remember is that this is not about you. By "this", I mean the experience someone else is having at the end of their life. Someone else is having the experience, and they are counting on YOU to help provide the support and comfort they need to make sure their death is done with dignity, kindness, comfort, compassion and care. So the very first thing you need to do is leave all of your "stuff" at the door. Shake it off, let it go and be fully and completely present for someone else. That is your gift to them; to walk into THEIR space fully and completely present.

I have walked into a patient's room and heard Brittney Spear's (for example) on the radio and I was pretty certain this wonderfully sweet ninety-five year old man did not want to hear that. I could be wrong, you can never assume someone else's musical taste, but for the most part I would say that he was not listening to that and probably doesn't want to. Our job is to be mindful of what he wants to hear, what sounds might bring him comfort and peace.

One of the first tips I was given, probably my first day of nursing school, was the importance of assessing the room when you first walk in. Whether this is a patient, a family member or a friend that you are caring for, assessing the room is important. Feel the energy, check on the family members, see if there might be someone else that could use your comfort and support as well. And truly look at the person laying in that bed; his eyes, his skin, his breathing, the temperature of the room, the amount of covers, or lack thereof... all of these things play into what he is experiencing.

Sometimes your patient can't verbalize his needs, so it is up to you to know what he needs and how you can help him. And check their toes... people have a habit of tucking the blankets in at the end of the bed... if you are dying, do you really want your toes all scrunched up at the end of the bed?? Let those toes wiggle and if it's not too cold, uncover them and let them breathe.

My biggest pet peeve is a dry mouth. A dry mouth, especially on someone who cannot verbally express their discomfort could cause agitation and restlessness. A quick swish of a mouth sponge, a drop of water on a tongue, the separation of the teeth against the gums... is like a mouth hug. Never leave your person with a dry mouth... it just isn't kind.

The best thing you can do for someone else is to make this about him or her and to remind him or her that they matter. This is NOT about you, and the more you acknowledge that, the more selfless you become.

Death And Religion

When you or someone you love begins hospice care, it comes with a team of amazing humans who provide comfort and support at the end of life. You will usually have a doctor, nurse, social worker, spiritual counselor, home health aid and a volunteer. The one I think that receives the most resistance is the spiritual counselor and it is usually because the patient already has a spiritual practice and doesn't feel they need more than that, or, they don't practice any particular faith and might not even believe in it at all. Some might have had a bad experience with a chaplain before, or are afraid they will only talk about Jesus or God, which for them, doesn't resonate. We respect their wishes and never push anything they are not comfortable with, however I do find myself taking a little extra time explaining that their role is not to impose their faith on you, but to instead be fully present for you while you work through the mysteries of the journey toward the end of life, spiritually or otherwise. I think of them as a spiritual guide, which helps to unravel some of the greatest curiosities that people face as they near death.

I once had a patient who as a child, had been forced to practice a religion that she did not understand. She was forced to say prayers she didn't believe and was told most of her young life that if she didn't follow this particular path, she would go to Hell. As an adult, she chose to walk away from the faith her family clung tightly to and in the process she lost her family. When she was diagnosed and given months or less to live, she accepted the care team, and refused the spiritual counselor, despite the multiple times I tried to sway her to at the very least, accept one visit.

We talked almost daily as she neared her last few days, and one day she asked me, "am I going to Hell"? She proceeded to tell me that her sister had called her earlier that day; they hadn't talked in years. She told her sister that she was going to die soon and asked her if she would come see her. Her sister told her no, that she was still standing strong with their parents and could not have a relationship with her as long as she continued to betray their faith. She told her that the reason she called was because she knew she was dying and wanted her to know that if she did not find faith now she would never go to Heaven.

It was very hard for me to not react, and to not come from a place of how this affected me personally. The truth is, I was so angry inside I wanted to call her myself and tell her what I thought. I was raised Catholic, my aunt is a nun and I still know all the words to several of the prayers. But as I aged, I found myself not having a connection to Catholicism, and really unsure of what I believe in, or what I needed in my life spiritually. I went to numerous churches, I spoke to people of many different faiths and I found myself embracing a variety of beliefs and being open and accepting to most of them.

At the time my patient asked me that question, I knew she only had hours to days left, and my answer needed to be one that could bring her comfort and relieve her from the feelings she was having. So I told her my truth; which I know might not be one held by all who read my blog. But I had to be honest, otherwise I think she would have seen through it and that could have added to the struggle she was already having after hearing her sisters words.

I said, "I am not 100% certain there is a Heaven or a Hell, nor am I convinced that dedicating your life to a specific faith, or not, will determine where you go when you die. What I do believe, and what I have seen in my work, is that those who do practice seem to have achieved comfort, and peace with their end. I see families pray, I see rosaries and crosses, and I hear prayers of all denominations and the peace it brings is lovely. I have seen someone who doesn't practice any faith, who has never prayed, and who might not believe, welcome the prayers of others and find true comfort from that. And I have known patient's that did not have, or want or need any spiritual support, and yet were completely at peace with where they were in their process and where they might be going after they die.

I believe that wherever I go when I die, I will be reunited with people who have passed, it will be beautiful and I will be strong, and healthy and have the ability to somehow look down upon those I left behind and watch over them. I do not believe I will go to Hell because I haven't made a commitment to anything in particular, and while I know I haven't always been kind, and I've told a lie or six, there is no higher power that would punish me for being human. So my answer is no, I do not think you are going to Hell. I think you are going somewhere beautiful, where you are surrounded by kindness and love". When I finished, I was afraid I might have said too much, or insinuated my own opinions inappropriately. But instead, she reached out and hugged me tightly, taking her time to let me go. I could feel her tears fall on to my shoulders, and could hear her sobs in my ear. She just kept saying "thank you" over and over.

I encouraged her to let me call one of our spiritual counselors to come visit her. I assured her that this person would simply sit with her, listen to her and provide comfort and support in whatever way she needed. It was at this time when I truly started to understand the role of our spiritual counselors and the benefits our patients and families receive from them. Their calming presence and ability to respect all wishes and ways of viewing life creates a safe place to help someone navigate through questions and concerns they might have relative to the end of life and what that might mean to each human uniquely.

That evening one of the spiritual counselors sat with her. She told me later that it was one of the most enlightening conversations she has ever had. She felt safe to reveal her own personal fears and even some regrets she didn't realize she had until she started to talk about them. She admitted that facing her own mortality, and subsequent death was powerful and scary and initially she felt alone and afraid, but after talking to the counselor, she felt the freedom to go in peace and was no longer fearful.

My feeling is this; death is hard on everyone regardless of whether you go to church every Sunday, meditate in the woods, or hike the highest mountains to achieve some semblance of inner peace. My work has given me the privilege of experiencing many different spiritual traditions and I am very thankful for that because it inspires me and opens my mind in a deep and powerful way. I do not think it is our place to inflict our own personal beliefs onto someone who is not open to receiving them. Religion is a personal and sometimes private choice and I think we should respect one another for our differences, even when it might be something we absolutely cannot entertain. And at the end of life, it is not kind to tell someone they will go to Hell if they do not pray or believe in what YOU feel is appropriate. Think about the words you might say to someone, especially in their last hours, and ask yourself, "will this provide comfort?" and if not, don't say them. Sometimes it's best to say nothing at all.

I Am Not An Angel

When someone asks you what you do and you tell them you are a hospice nurse, you always hear, "that must be so hard, how can you do that work every single day?" and there is also the "you must be an angel", which I struggle with. I am not an angel and while I appreciate the sentiment, the truth is, I am just a human who found her passion. But the fair question is; how can we do this work every single day?

I can remember a day like that very well. In the midst of having 5 patients to see, someone very dear to me fell and was taken to the hospital and declined quickly. Her family has become my family and I love them all very much. I wanted to be there for them, I wanted to help them. This is what I do, this is where I thrive, and I knew I could help them. BUT! I had five patients to see and my work had to be done first. I had two patients that were actively dying, I had another that took an hour to relieve her pain, I had a family member that was forty-five minutes late showing up to meet me and I had one that took me almost an hour to get to because of traffic. I felt like everything was against me being there for my friends (which I think of as family). All of this and the fact that I hadn't eaten anything all day, I was hot and sweaty and started to smell kind of yucky AND I HADN'T HAD A CHANCE TO PEE, put me in a very foul mood. But I finally finished and was able to be present at the bedside of a woman that was having a tough time and with a family I loved and it felt good to be there. I even put aside the fact that I still had five patients to chart for!!

Just as we were figuring out a plan for her and medications were being administered, I received a call from my office asking me to see another patient. This would be number six. We were short staffed and the family member was anxious, upset and needed us NOW!! I didn't want to go; I wanted to stay right where I was. I didn't want to be a nurse at that moment; I wanted to be a human having a difficult time knowing someone I love was hurting. But I said yes.

It took me forty minutes to get there; twice on the way I was called to ask my eta, which only infuriated me more. The second call was by our triage nurse, also frustrated because she was the one getting all the calls. I freaked out, I cried, I vented, and she listened. She stayed calm and she provided me with support.

I walked up to the door of my patient. I was hot, sweaty, starving and my eyes stung from crying and I shook it off. By the time I was inside with the husband and daughter, I was 100% hospice nurse. I provided them with comfort, support and active listening. I apologized for taking so long to get there. I relieved their wife/mother's pain. And I assured them that should her condition change during the night; we were just a phone call away. I was given hugs and "thank you's" when I left.

I am not an angel, nor am I a super human. Some days though, it feels like that is what is expected of us. We carry a lot of responsibility on our shoulders; working in hospice is hard. I had a tough day. I pushed myself too hard and I did NOT do any self-care.

When I got home I ate something and then I sat on the couch to start my charting for now six patients. But first I checked on my friends to see how they were doing and I checked in with the nurse who is caring for my friend/family member and made sure all was being well handled for her (and it was), I sent a "thank you" to the triage nurse who listened to me, and then I charted. Once I was done I took a nice long walk outside and I breathed in fresh air and gave myself a pat on the back and said "you did good today girl"... because sometimes that is all we need... a little pat on the back.

Some days are tough and I do wonder how the heck I can continue to do this work. That particular day was tough and I think it was really because I had something personal going on, somewhere else I wanted to be. I felt torn, I felt guilty, and I felt frustrated. But when I woke up the next morning, I felt good about myself, my work, the job I had done, despite it all, and I was ready for the new day and what it might bring. Before I headed out, I reminded myself; I will eat and I will pee and I should probably bring some deodorant with me. LOL

Most days are lovely, wonderful days. Some days are hard and difficult days. I am grateful for them all because all of this is what molds me into the human I am becoming and I love watching myself evolve and grow. But I have to remind myself that I am only human...

Take care of yourself... today and every day. YOU MATTER and someone needs you!! xo

Ativan, Morphine, Methadone OH MY!

If I could have my choice, I would have a death that was entirely comforted by compassionate and loving tactile stimuli, but the truth is, we almost always need the medications at the end of life. One of the struggles we often face is fear of the medications, especially Morphine or Methadone. People hear these words and they think addiction or death, as though, regardless of the terminal diagnosis, those medications will cause a death faster. Some families refuse them completely.

I had a patient many years ago, she was in her eighties and her main struggle was shortness of breath. The family was very against medication and wanted only to pray at the bedside to relieve her of her suffering. While I respected their faith, I asked her son to please allow me to give just a small dose of Morphine. I explained the benefits and the comfort I truly felt it would bring her. He refused, but in the same breath he kept saying to me, with his eyes filled with tears, "help my mom, please help my mom". He and his brother were the decision makers, but his brother was in Japan and he could not make any decisions without him. I climbed up in the bed with her, and I sat behind her to hold her as upright as I could and I too prayed that this would help, but I knew I couldn't help her and my own eyes filled with tears. I climbed off the bed and I looked him in the eyes and I sad, "I am going to the med cart and I am going to get a very small amount of Morphine and I am going to bring it back here. While I am gone, please call your brother, and let him know that I can help her but I need you to trust me." Knowing there was still a chance they would refuse and I needed to respect that, I went to the med cart and with shaking hands, I filled a syringe with only 5mg of Morphine and I walked back into their room. Her son looked at me and said, "We trust you".

I gave his mother Morphine and her breathing was calmed. This was a good day, and I was so thankful they agreed. I don't want to come off as a medication pusher but sometimes; these medications are the difference between a death with suffering and a death with peace.

People are afraid of medication and I get that. Before I became a nurse, I would have never thought that Methadone could bring as much relief as it does, because I can't help but equate it to the devastating addictions and/or deaths that it can provoke. The purpose and the outcome are different when administering medications to someone healthy vs. someone at the end of their life.

We spend a lot of time with families educating them about each medication, explaining how they provide relief and comfort, and reassuring them that the doses we administer are not going to hasten their death. Education is a powerful tool. If used correctly, it can ease the fear that many people experience relative to the medications we use. Another fear is addiction, I can't count how many times I have been asked, "will he/she become addicted"? While I never entertain that worry, their concern and their fear is real. I reassure them that becoming addicted is not a concern they need to have. I can say this with confidence because I know their end is near and these medications will only bring relief.

As clinicians, we understand the method of action for the medications we use, we know their benefits, we are usually prepared for their side effects and we have become almost immune to the fear of them. But that doesn't make it okay to downplay someone else's fear and I truly believe if we take the time to educate and reassure them about the medications we would like to administer, we can relieve their fear rather quickly.

I had a patient once tell me that Morphine was like a thick velvet blanket, that when given, will slowly flow through the body with comfort and softness, finding the places that ache the most, and sink deep into them until they are gone. I use this analogy often. I also like to say things like "Morphine and Lorazepam are good friends, they play nicely together" because people panic when we want to give more than one medication at a time. But at the end of the day, whether it is said straight forward or warm and fuzzy, all that really matters is that the family trusts you to administer whatever medication you feel will reduce pain and suffering.

It is all about trust. Our first responsibility with a patient and their family is to build trust. Once we establish that, and are able to break down some of the walls, we can work together to ensure a softer landing, but in order to do that we need to communicate, educate and respect the fears our patient's and families might have.

Self Care

This work is hard. In one day I could see one patient who is actively dying and have to tell the family there are only hours to days left, then I go to see another patient who's pain is 10/10 and I struggle with relieving him but do whatever I can until I do, and then I can walk into a home minutes before a patient takes his last breath and I need to let this family know that all they have is right this second to come to the bedside and say their final goodbyes and I watch as his breaths slow and the family realizes that "this is it" and he passes away. And no matter how prepared they are, that last breath is a shock and their pain is real. I go straight into the role of providing comfort and support to those at the bedside. I give them all of me. And by the end of that day... I am exhausted; emotionally and physically exhausted. And the next day, I do it all over again. Because that is how it's done in hospice.

Rarely does anyone ask me how my day is, because they are afraid I am really going to tell them. My days are difficult. I cry A LOT. And yet I still find the strength to move forward and give just as much to the family I see next, as the one I just left. I absolutely 100% love my job. I love doing hospice work. But!! If we do not take care of ourselves we will burn out and we will not be able to give what we give. We absolutely must take care of ourselves. For me it is finding someone to talk to, whether it is someone I work with or random strangers on a hospice FB page. But I need to talk about it. Writing about it helps me as well.

Writing "Soft Landing" was such an incredible form of therapy for me, that when I published it and was done, I felt a sense of loss. So I started on my next book, which is what you are reading now. I also paint, and I take walks, lots of walks. The other thing I have done is I have created a "grief bowl" which was given to me by a wonderful Shaman named Linda Fitch. In this bowl I have placed two rose quartz hearts and when I have had a tough day, I hold onto those hearts and I think about the patient I was with, the people who love them, the work I did and I let it go and sometimes I sit and cry. And then I place the hearts in the bowl until the next time... and there are a lot of "next times". That grief bowl helps me. I suggest you find a ritual that is yours specifically, something sacred and special that heals you within. But whatever you do, however you find your peace, take care of you always. You do not do this job alone, there is a team of people in hospice that are there for you as well as the patient and family, you just have to go to them. It is okay to admit that you struggle with all the loss and all the death and all of the ache and pain you see every single day.

You are a lovely human for what you do... hold that in your heart. Know that you do beautiful work. But please, don't forget to take care of you!!! xoxox

It Takes A Village

As a nurse, one of the most important lessons I have learned in hospice is the importance of the team that you share your patient with. I didn't always play nice with others, in fact to be honest I didn't think I needed them and in many ways I became a little territorial with MY patients not understanding why the social worker or chaplain was encroaching on MY time with MY patient. I know... how selfish right? And don't I always say, "this isn't about you"? Sometimes I need to follow my own advice!!!

This has since changed significantly. Each patient is assigned a doctor, a nurse, a spiritual counselor, a social worker, a home health aid and sometimes, if they are lucky, a volunteer. Each one of these team members brings something unique and valuable to the care of the patient, but also to the fluidity of each situation. Death is not predictable, how someone goes through their process is not predictable. How a family member or friend works through their loss is not predictable. The team works together to find the best way to help make the struggle a little less painful or difficult.

Over the years I have come to learn the vast amount of information each member of the team brings, and I have learned to count on them; I go to them for answers, because I have learned... I do not have them all!!! I have also gone to them for help for myself; for comfort, for support, for guidance and clarity. I need this team, as much as the patient and family do.

The home health aids are lovely, their work, is lovely. They are more up close and personal with each patient than most members of the team. They have a special kind of sensitivity and kindness that makes our patients feel safe. If you are a caregiver, CNA or HHA, I say THANK YOU!!!

My favorite members of the team are the volunteers. They are givers of the truest sense of the word, and so incredibly unselfishly. They don't do this for financial reasons or for accolades; in fact I think most prefer to fly a little under the radar. But their presence and gentle nature and total commitment to our patients is deep and beautiful and amazing and I love them. I truly love them! If you are a volunteer, please know that I appreciate you, more than you will ever know.

Embrace the team. Appreciate the team. Support the team. Count on the team.

End of Life Option Act (EOLOA)
Death With Dignity
Medical Aid In Dying

As a hospice nurse, I have seen, understandably, a LOT of death. I have been blessed to witness beautiful, peaceful deaths and that is what I strive for with every patient. Some patient's, however have had a very difficult time and pain was unmanageable. Sometimes, no amount of medication brings relief. I struggle with this.

I had a patient that had severe pain and shortness of breath; nothing I did brought her comfort, and despite how many I tried, no medications reduced her suffering. When the EOLOA was first approved in California, it was the first time I saw her have some semblance of hope. While her diagnosis was terminal, there was no certainty of the timing, which meant however many days, weeks or months she had left, she would be in pain. This was not the way she wanted to live her last days of life. EOLOA allowed her to have a choice to end her pain with dignity.

I was there the day she did this. My heart was sad because I had grown very fond of her, but I knew, this was the kindest way for her to go and she would no longer feel pain and that was all I wanted for her. Hers was a beautiful death, surrounded by people she loved, with Buddhist prayers and chanting. I felt extremely honored to have been asked to be there that day.

I respect people who do not support EOLOA. I have no intention of changing your mind; that is not for me to do. But at the very least, remove yourself from the equation and imagine a terminally ill person, who is riddled with pain and struggles for breath. Someone has to change their diapers and bathe them because they do not have the strength or energy to do it any more. They are dying, and this won't change, but their death will be long, drawn out and painful.

Doesn't this patient deserve the chance to at the very least, choose to shorten the timing of the inevitable and have it be kinder, gentler and bring them peace?

This isn't about us. This is their experience and if this is something they choose, the best thing we can do is support them, be there for them and not judge or punish them. I have been present for many EOLOA deaths; the moment they take the glass in their hands and swallow down the medications is the moment you know, that they know... their pain and suffering will be over.

Death Happens

You would think working in hospice you would become less surprised by the ache and pain you see others experience when death is verified. I saw a patient once, she was in her late 60's and it was very clear to me that she was starting her process and if I was to guess, I would say she was hours away from taking her last breath.

Her husband of fifty-four years was not ready to give up hope, he was not willing to believe that her time was up and refused to have "that" discussion. When I arrived, she was experiencing pain, but it was not clear where from. I feel confident that her whole body was riddled in pain. I desperately wanted to give her something; my medication of choice was Morphine. He refused initially because he was absolutely certain it was the "death medication" and if she was being given that, it was the admission that death was near. He wanted nothing to do with anything that didn't hold out hope.

I am sure many of you in hospice have had the conversations about Morphine; people are frightened... it has a scary and negative connotation and most people think it will cause addiction or death. I had a patient once that told me he thought of morphine as a velvet blanket that once taken, feels as though it wraps around you, comforting all the places that ache and makes you feel cozy and safe. This is the explanation I give to many and it is the one I gave to him. He finally gave in and Morphine was administered. It took about twenty minutes before I could see she was more relaxed. I assured him that he could call our after-hours line if she was not relieved of her pain and that I would make sure a nurse was scheduled the next day to come back and check on her.

I was scheduled to visit him that next day. About fifteen minutes prior to me heading there, I received a call that he thought she had passed and wanted to call 911 and have someone resuscitate her and make her better. The triage nurse told him I was on my way and asked him to please wait. I drove so fast to get there, I was certain I would get pulled over, in fact I had decided on my route that if that happened, I would just keep going until I got there and deal with it when we arrived. Because I knew, this husband needed me NOW and nothing was going to get in my way.

When I walked in the door, he was standing there in the living room, his eyes so red and puffy they were hard to see. "She died Gabby. She died. She stopped breathing. What happened?" And I went to him and hugged him tight and asked to see her to make sure. I walked over to her bedside and I knew. But I needed to go through the proper steps and listen for a heartbeat and feel a pulse. As I placed my stethoscope against her chest I took in a deep breath as I prepared myself to turn around and give him the news he never wanted to hear. I know he was hoping that I would say something else, to tell him that he was wrong and she was just deeply sleeping. I took my stethoscope and slowly put it over my head and on my shoulders and I very slowly turned to face him. "I'm so sorry, she passed" and I reached for him to hug him. I could feel his tears soak through my scrubs. I could feel his heart break. And while I knew I was not responsible, I was the one that gave the news and for a brief second I really, really hated my job. I cried as I watched him call his kids.

I convinced him to help me bathe and change her before their kids arrived. I changed her clothes and brushed her hair and I repositioned her in such a way that she looked beautiful and at peace. I asked him to go out to the garden and pick a flower for her to hold. He walked in with a blue hydrangea and asked, "is this one okay"? I took the flower and tucked it tightly in her hands that were carefully placed in her lap. He said, "she looks so beautiful". We sat at her bedside for about fifteen minutes as he told me about their life and their love.

His kids arrived while I was still there, as did friends and family that rushed over the minute they heard. News spread fast and he was supported and loved by many. Before I left I reminded him what a beautiful job he did caring for her. He asked how it happened so fast; he needed answers. I tried to use all the right words to help him to understand that while his hope and faith for her to recover was strong, her diagnosis was stronger and it had a mind of its own. I assured him that his care allowed her a longer time than was probably expected and he should hold that close to his heart.

I walked out and got into my car and drove about 30 feet to a shady spot under a tree and I cried. As I say often, I see death but I also see love, deep, amazing, and beautiful love. I reminded him before I left that some people in their entire lifetime never feel the love he had for her and she was blessed to have that. He told me he was too.

Bedside Manner

When someone is lying in a bed and they are unable to verbalize how they are feeling or what they might need, that is the most important time for you to be sensitive, considerate and kind.

Please do not do anything without telling them first, they deserve to be included in anything that you might be doing to or for them. Talk to them before you clean their mouth, or change their brief or raise or lower their bed. Let them know you are about to touch them. It's already scary enough going through their dying process, but can you imagine laying in a bed, without a voice, eyes are closed and someone comes along and shoves a cotton swab in your mouth, or suddenly removes your pillow or worse... puts medication in your mouth... none of which without warning?!?!? Talk to them, tell them what you are about to do; this is their body; ask permission first, they have the right to be asked first, or at the very least, told.

The liquid medications used most frequently in my experience have been Morphine, Lorazepam, Haloperidol and Methadone, most of which absorb through the mucus membranes, except for Morphine, which has to be swallowed. These medications are bitter and don't taste good. I have learned that putting these medications in a moist mouth is less yucky than a dry mouth. If you take a syringe and drop one or two drops of water on the tongue before giving the medication, it's just a little easier for them. BUT!!! And don't forget this part: tell them first! Just because they can't verbalize, and might be sedated, does not mean they do not have feelings and cannot be startled or scared. Always tell them first when you are about to put something in their mouth. If you massage the cheeks, it helps the medication absorb a little easier. Sometimes a little trickles down their throat and causes them to cough; elevate their head a little more and reassure them you are there and it's okay and relieve them of the fear that they might be choking. I like to reach my arm under their pillow, getting their head into the curve of my arm (near the elbow) and slightly lift their head up just enough to help them get the medications down, without having them pool or settle in the throat and cause that really uncomfortable feeling. Be gentle, be kind, take your time... don't rush patient care... EVER! When someone is lying in a bed and they are unable to verbalize how they are feeling or what they might need, that is the most important time for you to be sensitive, considerate and kind.

Mouth care is a wonderful gift for someone lying in a bed, especially for those who cannot tell you how they feel. Don't do mouth care after you have given medication though, wait at least forty-five minutes to make sure it's been absorbed. Mouth care before medication though, is lovely!!! Get that sponge in there, separate the teeth and gums, and moisten their tongue. Trust me... they will love this!!!

A few tips when providing cooling measures... a cool cloth on a warm head is lovely, do it and do it often BUT.... DON'T LEAVE IT THERE! It drives me insane to walk into a room and see someone lying there with a washcloth on their head that I know, has been there awhile. Remember, a cool cloth on a warm head becomes a warm heavy cloth and that does not feel good. Gently dab the cloth on the forehead, the cheeks, the back off the neck, and over the eyes. Not both eyes at the same time though, that can be claustrophobic, dab one eye and then the other. And don't forget to tell them what you are doing the entire time. Medications tend to make eyes and cheeks hot, and that cool cloth is a gift from you they will be so appreciative for. If they have an oxygen cannula on, remember to periodically raise and lower the tubing from where it rests on the cheeks, it tends to dig deep into their skin and is uncomfortable.

Before I get off my "bedside manner soap box" I want to tell you one more pet peeve, although not the last I am sure... Do not turn lights on that will shine right into someone's eyes without at least telling them first, and if you can provide care without that light, do it!!! In general no one wants light shining in their eyes but someone lying in a hospital bed, nearing the end of life, is more sensitive, more fragile and those lights can be blinding and will sting.

Be considerate and kind always... to your patients, to yourself and to others!

Work/Life Balance

I struggle with saying "no". I am THAT nurse; the one that will agree to see another patient after I have already seen five. Or work the weekend shifts, or stay late or sit at the bedside with the family until the last breaths are taken. I have a hard time leaving a family when I know someone only has a short time left. BUT! I have finally come to realize that I cannot do my job the way I want to, I cannot be the nurse I want to be AND I cannot give completely to a patient or their family if I have burnt my candles at both ends.

Hospice nursing/end of life care requires you to be fully present for someone else at one of the most difficult times of his or her lives. How can you possibly commit to that if you are not balancing work and life? What does that mean exactly? It means finding balance between your work and your private life but most importantly, HAVING A PRIVATE LIFE. Setting boundaries, taking breaks, and knowing when to turn off the job is key. I am still working on that. If I have a patient who is actively dying, I will check the after hours reports to see if they have passed. I try not to, but I cannot just shut them off. I didn't realize just how badly I needed to practice this until my candle became a puddle of wax and I was exhausted.

I am learning to say "no", to slow down and take my time with each patient and to make sure that I take care of me in the process. I am not good at it, this will be a daily practice for me and I am a constant work in process. BUT! I am allowing the fear of losing my love for this work to be my guide. I don't want my sparkle to dull; I don't want to carry anger or frustration into my patient's home. I want to take time to breathe, to meditate, to stretch and practice the self-care I mention in many of my blog postings. I want to be physically, mentally and emotionally ready to provide the very best care to my patients and their families. I want to always find sparkle in what I do, and the best way is to find balance between work and play.

You don't wear a cape; you are not a super human. I am NOT a super human. I am just a human who truly loves what I do... with a desire to do it as long as I am able. So I will say this now... for all of you to hear... from this moment forward, I will find balance between work and my personal life. I will shut my phone off. I will stop reading all the emails when I am off the clock. I will sleep in, I will visit with family and friends, I will laugh and I will dance and I will play. All of this I will do because I want to be fully present for our patient's; I want to give them the very best version of me.

Charting. (*This one is for the Clinicians*)

This is definitely on my top five list of things I have so much to say about!! After a long day of seeing patients, barely taking a break to eat or pee, remembering to order medications/supplies, possibly getting new medication/treatment orders from the MD... charting is the thing most of us dread doing. BUT it is one of the most important things we do for so many reasons.

Nothing frustrates me more than preparing to see a patient, especially for the first time, and not finding any current documentation in their chart. This is unacceptable to me. It's bad enough to see minimal information documented but to not even have the last visit started makes me scream. Internally. Oh!! And don't get me started on things that are left out of the documentation.

If you know me, you know my charting is always way too long and wordy. I understand this and I do not expect others to follow suit. But I see documentation as a road map of the decline of the patient. In my first days of nursing school, we were told to write our documentation with the idea that many years down the road, for whatever reason, someone may be looking at your charting. Your job, is to make sure there is no need for questions, because you made yourself very clear AND created a detailed picture of what that patient was experiencing during your visit. Write everything you can so no one needs to question you.

This is what I think about when I chart; I think about WHO will read it. I start with the MD/NP and what information I think they would want to know. I think about the case manager or other nurses that might see this patient. I think about the social worker and the chaplains and make sure I incorporate any dynamics or spiritual questions/concerns. I also think about the caregivers, home health aids and volunteers.

I always include intake/output, emotional state, pain level, skin changes, family dynamics, near death awareness/concerns and how quickly their decline might be. If the patient is in pain and has been taking additional pain meds, or increased PRN's, I include date/time/dose, so that the MD/CM can keep track. I also include areas of sensitivity, for instance; "left sided weakness", or "don't touch right shoulder". Provide the information that will best describe what the patient is currently experiencing, but also what will help those seeing the patient after you. Your words can determine the care that patient receives after you. You can help make sure they are tended to appropriately, kindly and considerately.

Imagine you saw a patient and there was a significant decline, or medication change, or information you gave the family that was valuable and important but you didn't document after your visit. And then something happens, shortly after you left, so they called the after-hours/triage nurse to discuss it. The person answering the phone goes to that patient's chart and does not see anything, has nothing to go on. This is not fair to the triage nurse, the family member or the patient.

Charting is important!! Do it as soon after your visit as you can and do it with thought and consideration!!! And if you don't have the time right after your visits, at the very least, add the significant stuff in the narrative so there is something there. I get it, the days are long and it's really hard to chart after your visit, but this isn't about you. This is about the care our patient's receive and that is our responsibility.

This Time It's Personal

When I was seventeen I dated a guy whose mother I rubbed the wrong way. The midnight intoxicated teenage calls to him didn't help. I got a lecture or two about the time I was calling, and was encouraged not to do it again (I believe I was not a good listener and did it again, and again). I feel blessed that almost forty years later this same family became my family and my love for them is real. I have a different relationship with each member of the family and I cherish each one of them for their differences and the gifts each bring into my life.

Recently that same woman I annoyed as a teenager became one of our patient's and I found myself being torn between being a hospice nurse and a friend. This was a new experience for me. I found myself almost unsure of what to do or what to say or how best to provide comfort and care for people I love. We ended up taking her to our hospice house, which was such a blessing for her and her family. I honestly didn't need to do anything, I just felt this need to do everything and this was difficult for me. I was able to check in with the staff, suggest increased medications or at least collaborate with them as we moved forward, but the truth is, they did just fine without me and they did not need me to help. This too was hard for me. I didn't have a place and I struggled with this.

I found that the best thing I could do, was to educate the family on what was to be expected, support them as her condition changed and alert them as she declined further and became imminent. These are people I love so much and each was going thorough their own way of working through this experience. They are private people, not terribly emotional and certainly do not throw their emotions out for all to see. I am the exact opposite, so my additional struggle was to hold back from forcing them to express feelings they preferred to keep to themselves.

The one thing I did, which was private, lovely and special for all who participated, was to take a photo of each one holding her hand before she passed. I don't think they would have done that on their own so I am glad to have encouraged that.

Once again I am reminded that this is not about me, which also includes accepting and respecting how other people deal with death and dying, even people you love and care for personally. I was honored to share in the care of this woman. I was in awe of the staff and the wonderful job they did. And I felt lucky to be at the bedside with the family as we all said goodbye to the woman responsible for bringing us all together. These are my friends, and they are my family... I will keep them forever.

It's Okay To Sing Off Key

I have been writing this in my head since the day she arrived, because the moment I met her, I knew immediately there was a special place in my heart that had been saved for her. She was in her forties', and by age she was an adult, but she was more like a child in her thoughts, in what little words she was able to verbalize and in her simple joys and pleasures that brought a smile to her absolutely beautiful face. Her eyes were a pale blue that opened wide when she showed happiness, and "happiness" was brought on by her family, memories of friends she made at her previous care facility and children's nursery rhymes and songs.

When I first sat down with her father and her twin sisters, who were younger than her, I knew this was a person who was loved very much. The attention to detail in the care provided her by this family is something all should be lucky enough to experience. While I know hospice, and I know patient care and I feel confident about what I do for someone at the end of life, I do not pretend to know a patient more than their family or friends, or even the people who cared for them before they came to us. So I welcome their knowledge, their opinions, their thoughts and their suggestions. This was a perfect example of that. Her younger sisters knew her very well and were able to convey to us the best way to care for her. She would require us to be sensitive to movement, sound, and touch.

My first meeting with her was one I will carry with me for the rest of my life. She struggled with putting words together and forming sentences, but she was able to say my name and when I sang nursery songs to her, she sang with me and my heart smiled huge. I was in awe of the gentle way her sisters cared for her, the love they have for her is something rare, deep and beautiful. I found myself drawn to this family for many different reasons and I visited with them and their sister, our patient, quite frequently throughout each day she was with us. And when the family stepped away, I would sit at her bedside.

When I was a little kid, I wanted to sing but couldn't carry a tune. I couldn't even sing "happy birthday" without being told it was best I didn't sing. I remember one Christmas; our school was putting on a musical performance. I wasn't allowed to sing, and instead was put on set building, but I told my mom I was going to sing "The Little Drummer Boy". The night of the performance, my mom was out in the audience and I was in the back helping with sets. When "my" song was about to start, I ran out to the stage and climbed up onto the back riser and joined the group. I mouthed all the words. I got in trouble that night by my teacher, made fun of by the other students and told I was an embarrassment by my mother. I never sang out loud again and even now, I usually just mouth the words to "Happy Birthday".

But at her bedside, I sang "twinkle, twinkle little star" over and over and I didn't care who heard me, and when she was able to join in I felt so much joy in my heart. I sang every nursery rhyme I could remember. Some days it was just she and I, some days I sang with her sisters and one day her dad joined in. And then the days moved along and she couldn't sing back, but I continued singing to her, because I knew it brought her joy. On her last day with us, I was able to go and visit her. I sat at her bedside with her sister and together we sang one last round of "twinkle, twinkle".

I know she had good care by our team, I know we reduced her pain and discomfort and I know we gave her family a place to come to be at her bedside, to feel supported and to feel confident that someone they loved was being treated well. But I wonder if they know what they did for us, and for the purpose of this story, what they did for me. They all brought me joy, they reminded me to appreciate the simplest of things, and they let me know it was okay to sing off key. I will remember this sweet soul always.

We bathed her, we braided her hair, and we placed a white rose in her hands. As she was wheeled out to the car, we sprinkled rose petals on her and sang "twinkle, twinkle". No more sleeps sweet girl, but no more pain either.

Life Is Fragile And Precious

We had a patient pass recently; it happened while I had stepped out for a bit and when I walked in the door, I was told he was gone. He was only with us two days, I hadn't become close to him, I hadn't really spent much time with him at all, but when I walked in the door of his room to say goodbye, I had this almost profound experience. I looked at him lying in the bed and I thought to myself, "he's gone" and wondered for a second why this hadn't happened to me before. I had to question myself... had I become so numb to death that death itself didn't affect me any more?

I stood next to his bed and I took his hand in mine and held it; it was so cold. I started to talk to him; I told him I hoped we had provided good care, that I was sorry his last few days were such a struggle and I hoped that wherever his journey took him, it was safe, peaceful, and beautiful. And for a few moments I felt sadness. It was sadness for the loss of a life, about his pain and struggle in his last few days and the knowing of his own pain and struggle and how hard that must have been for him.

We filled our ceremonial bowl with lavender water and fresh roses and we placed washcloths in it until they were soaked with the calming aroma. We put candles around his room. I watched and listened as Khristian, another nurse, spoke eloquently and kindly about him and extended such sensitivity to his family. I handed his sister and his son the scented washcloths and gave them time to gently wash his hands, his feet and his face. I felt deeply touched by this ritual as I watched, and was almost surprised by how much it affected me. I have participated in many of these beautiful baths, but was taken aback by the way it was affecting me this time.

After we walked him out to the car and said goodbye to his son and his sister, I went back into his room. I opened the doors to the patio and felt this swish of wind go past me, as though someone had walked by me. But no one was there. I walked outside on to the patio and I took in the smell of the rose bushes, the sounds of the birds, the warmth of the sun and the power of the sky above me and thought to myself how happy I am to be alive and I felt this deeper appreciation for my life and all the wonderfulness of it all. I took it all in and I took several deep breaths to allow it to consume me completely.

I am not sure why his death affected me so deeply; perhaps it was the gentle reminder I needed to stay focused on the present, to embrace each moment, to feel gratitude for life and to appreciate each human as they go through their process. This doesn't mean I don't, but perhaps I have allowed my own distractions to get in the way a bit.

For the remainder of the day I felt as though I were walking a little less in a hurry, breathing a little less quickly, and feeling such peace and joy within. I feel like my eyes and my heart were opened just a tiny bit more. Life is fragile and precious, people are fragile and precious, and kindness and compassion are gifts we give one another but also to ourselves. Especially in this kind of work, but I think also in life, we have to breathe in beautiful and exhale gratitude. Be kind to each other. Be appreciative of life. Don't take anything for granted.

Never Apologize For Being Kind

I will never get tired of seeing people being kind to strangers, or just being kind in general. One day while working in our hospice house, the AC went out. Thankfully it wasn't a serious problem and it was a very easy fix but leading up to that is something that will stay in my heart always.

At 3:00pm, I called the Air Conditioning company who said they closed at 4:30pm and "IF" they could get someone to come out, it would be overtime. She didn't think she could find someone that late. I admit it; I played the "hospice" card and said we had patients and families that needed the air conditioning on as soon as possible. She promised to call me back to let me know if they were able to find someone. About thirty minutes later I received the call that someone would be there in 1-2 hours. I was just grateful someone was coming out, so I didn't ask any questions about the "who" or the "why" or the "how"

About 5:30pm a repairman showed up. We started talking and he told me that when he heard it was a hospice house, he offered to come despite the fact that he was already on his way home to be with his family. His mother-in-law passed away a few years ago and the hospice team that cared for her was so wonderful he wanted to give back. He knew our patients needed the AC and that was a priority for him. He fixed the problem and the air was on. He offered to stay until the house cooled to make sure everything was working okay. I offered him coffee, which he accepted. I offered to make it, but he said he saw the coffee maker at the coffee station and could make it himself. This kindness story doesn't stop here.

After about ten minutes, I could hear him talking so I went out to see whom he was talking to. The daughter of a patient was out in the dining area; she had come to the coffee station and was clearly crying. He saw her in tears, and asked if she was okay. She felt safe and comfortable with him, so shared her story. By the time I walked out, he was hugging her. She thanked him for the hug and as she passed by me to go sit with her mom, she said to me "he was so kind". When I went over to him, he immediately apologized for talking to her, he said she came up to him; he was worried that he had done something wrong. I reassured him that he did nothing wrong, that his heart is a beautiful heart and he was at the right place at the right time and provided her with exactly what she needed at the time. I walked him out to his truck and watched as he tried to wipe away a tear without me seeing. I put my arm on his shoulder and said, "I get it… it happens to me every day". He thanked me for what we do and left.

Shortly after that, the daughter he had spoken to earlier, came to apologize for "interfering" with our work that was being done, she said she was just so emotional and couldn't stop crying and he was so kind and supportive. Again, I had to say that you never have to apologize for being kind.

Be kind to others, it's easy to do
Be kind to others and they will be kind to you
Share you heart, lend an ear
Give a hug, comfort tears
Your kindness matters, it's a true gift indeed
Be kind to someone, when you see a need
Or just be kind in general, it comforts the soul
Days can be hard; pain takes a toll
Imagine if your kindness removed sadness or pain
Imagine the comfort that person would gain
Be kind to others… it's easy to do

It Doesn't Get Easier

Before I started my day, I called a family to let them know I would be there about noon. I left a voicemail. I was with another patient when the daughter called me back to say that noon was fine, but that they would be there all day and time was not a problem. (I repeat… time was not a problem.) These are words everyone takes such advantage of, and this time was no different.

While I was with a patient, my phone rang, I did not recognize the number and I never take calls when I am with a patient, but there was such urgency in the sound of the ring as though the universe was telling me I needed to take that call. So I did. It was the daughter calling me back, her mother's breathing had changed and she asked if I could come now. She was crying and while I didn't know how her mother was doing, I knew for sure her daughter needed support and reassurance, so I told her I would be there soon. I was already preparing to leave at the time of the call, so I grabbed my things and headed to see them.

When I walked up the doorstep, there was this feeling I had that told me things were not okay in that house; I felt the urge to cry but I had no idea why. I rang the doorbell and within half a second, I heard footsteps running towards the door. This lovely young woman opened the door; she was in her early twenties' I am guessing, eyes swollen and red from crying and she hugged me tight, thanking me for getting there so soon and said, "please come check on my mom". I just knew… even before I knew… and my heart ached.

When I walked into the room, I honestly thought she had passed, but I could still see a faint pulse in her neck and knew that while she was still breathing, it wouldn't be for long. I felt the need to give the family more time and told them they only had a few minutes, and to use this time to give her some more love and I stepped out of the room.

When I walked back in, I sat down on the floor next to the bed and I looked at her daughter and let her know she had taken her last breath. I wish so badly it wasn't me giving that message because the look in her eye's made every ounce of me want to cry. They were not prepared for this news, they didn't want to say goodbye, and they were not ready to let her go. Are we ever really ready to let someone go? Does it ever get easier? Why do people say things like "it will get easier"? No, it DOES NOT get easier on either end… the saying goodbye to someone, or telling someone they need to say goodbye. It does not get easier.

I let them have time with her and I waited outside on the couch. Her daughter came out to me in tears and sat next to me. I wrapped my arms around her and let her sit there with me and cry. She kept saying "why?" I wish so badly that I had the answer for that. I wish so badly I could fix her heart and make it ache less. But she wanted an answer; she needed me to say something. So I told her that while I was not practicing any specific faith, I do believe that wherever she goes, she will be without any pain or discomfort. And then I shared with her something I have always hoped to be true, which is what I feel about my sister when she passed away, and that is that she was so wonderful and so good and so giving, that she filled her role here, she did what she needed to do and now she is needed somewhere else to continue the gifts she gives. Her daughter said she agreed, that she did do "good" here. And she cried some more, and I held her longer.

Before I left, I pulled her daughter aside and reminded her what a beautiful job she did caring for her mother, that it was because of her that she was able to take her last breaths without any distress or struggle and that it was so peaceful and so incredibly gentle. I told her that her gift to her mother was her love and kindness and that she will always carry that with her.

And as I walked out to my car I started to cry... and I am crying now as I write this because it does not get easier. Loss is loss and pain is pain and when the heart aches... it just aches. And while I can go days or months without feeling sadness for my losses, it is days like this that they are brought up again. But then I smiled, because I got to remember about my sister and how good she was to me and how truly lucky I was to have her for the amount of time I did.

Saying goodbye doesn't get easier... and having to tell someone it's time to say goodbye doesn't get easier...

Start The Conversation

I walked into the room of a patient who was in a facility, at the same moment the floor nurse walked in to give medication. She walked up to him and squirted medication in his mouth. She did not let him know ahead of time, she did not do it with kindness or consideration and she did not stay long enough to even make sure he didn't choke. I was so disappointed in this care that I found myself filling up with anger.

Just because someone is non-responsive and near death does not take away the fact that they are still human and their experience is real, and difficult. At the very least, she could have said hello to him, let him know she was there and what she was doing. She could have talked to him while she was doing it. She could have dropped a little water on his tongue so the taste was less bitter. She could have stayed a moment to make sure he was okay. And she could have respected him and treated him with kindness but she did not.

So I have a confession; I tracked her down at the nurse's station and asked if I could talk with her. She immediately pointed to the patient binders and said I would find everything I needed there and started to walk away. I followed her, I asked her to please stop for a minute so we could talk. She said she was busy, and again started to walk away. By now I was just plain angry. So I yelled at her "hopefully you will treat the next person you see kinder than the one you just left" and I turned around and walked away. I could hear her coming up behind me and I won't lie, I was a little afraid.

But what happened after that was perfect for me and for her. She asked me what I meant and why I said that. I explained that her approach was cold and insensitive, that she didn't even let him know what she was doing. I explained that he still has feelings and especially because he is unable to verbalize his needs and his eyes are closed, he deserves kindness and consideration. I explained that coming up to someone like that could be scary. I explained that anyone lying in a bed nearing death is probably afraid and it is our job to be their advocate, to be kind and give them the consideration they deserve.

She started to cry. She had just recently graduated nursing school; there were a few hours of discussion about grief in school but nothing about hospice. (I remember this well). This was the first place that hired her so she took the job because she wanted to be a hospice nurse. She was hoping to be trained, educated and taught how to be a hospice nurse, but instead she was taught how to use the computer program, how to pass meds, where supplies were and whom the team was… but never was she taught anything about bedside care. I got it, I totally got it and I felt so bad for her. So I asked her when her break was and offered to sit with her during her break and help her as much as I could in 30 minutes.

We sat down together and talked hospice. It was a quick review but it started the conversation and it inspired her to want to learn more. She is not an unkind person; in fact as I started to talk to her, I realized how kind her heart was. This was someone who wanted to do a job she was totally unprepared for. And it reminded me how little education there is for people caring for someone at the end of life.

After that day, we would meet once a week for about an hour and there were multiple text conversations in between and I helped her; I guided, encouraged, inspired and supported her. About four months later, she called to tell me about a patient she had cared for that passed away with her at his bedside. She let me know that she was fully present for him, that she provided comfort, compassion and kindness and she assured me his landing was soft. I am so proud of her.

What if we all took time to educate those who want to learn? What if we shared our tools with others to help build them up? It doesn't have to be a nurse; it could be any human whose heart chooses to sit at the bedside of a dying patient. Let's work together to build our hospice community; this amazing community that does beautiful work can only get better if bigger. Let's make our community bigger!!!

Grief Is A Dance In Uncomfortable Shoes

Much like death, grief is not predictable. We do not grieve the same way, it doesn't happen on queue; there isn't a rulebook that says: "this is how you will feel and when". My father passed away over twenty years ago and I am only now truly feeling that loss. My sister passed away less than that, and my heart aches for her daily. Some people cry, some people hold it in, some people wonder why they don't feel a thing, and some wonder when the tears will stop and the pain will end.

I received a call from the husband of a patient I had that passed away a few years ago, to the day to be exact. I asked him how he was doing; he said he has good days and bad days. He talked about the changes in his life since she passed away; he finally started cooking again, he moved the furniture around, the cat finally sleeps with him now and the plant they grew from seed, that almost died when she got sick is blooming. He said, "life continues". It sounded so forced, as though he felt he was supposed to say it, supposed to go on and move forward. It sounded almost robotic. I don't think he has moved on, I don't think he has moved forward. I think he says all the things he thinks everyone wants to hear, but I get the feeling he is stuck in time, back to when he lost the love of his life and can't seem to get beyond that.

This got me thinking about death and life and life after death; and the difficulty each person has moving on. I move on, from one patient to the next; one mother, one father, one sister, one brother… so many deaths I can't even count them any more. But I don't forget. I too grieve; sometimes I grieve for the patient, sometimes for the people left behind, and sometimes I am reminded of my own personal losses that I have tucked deep inside until I remember again. Sometimes I cry, sometimes I smile, sometimes I am just grateful for the memories.

I think that is what grief is, at least for me. It is the reminder of someone we loved and lost. It is the memories we had, and the fact that we will not be able to make any more. If you have read my book or my previous blogs, you have heard me say this before; I have a favorite quote: "My memories say hello, they ask about you all the time". That is what grief is to me. It is missing the person I made so many memories with; from my parents, to my sister, to the many friends I have lost... I miss making memories with them. But again, I am so thankful I can remember.

I think moving forward I will continue to live a life of memory making. For my families, at their deepest time of loss, I will encourage them to remember and to move through their grief with whatever emotion comes their way. Some days will bring laughter, some days will bring tears, and some days will bring anger because they are no longer here but hopefully each day we will be reminded of the love we once had, the memories we made and the truly beautiful impact they had on our life.

Grief is a dance in uncomfortable shoes; we hear the music, we feel the need to move with it, but sometimes we are clumsy, we lose balance and we fall. And sometimes we glide gracefully, with ease. Just know... that it is also okay if you stand still for a bit and sway, just don't stop listening to the music.

Death Does Not Have A Time Clock

After spending many hours at the home of a patient who is actively dying and working with a family who is struggling with the difficult task of finding the words to say goodbye… I close the door and I walk away. It feels like time stops and seconds take minutes and walking to my car feels like crossing the finish line after doing a marathon. I am completely and totally spent. And the crazy thing about this is that I wake up every morning ready to do it again.

I never know what I have waiting for me on the other side of a door I am about to knock on. I have been called to see a patient who was actively dying and they lived two more weeks, and I have been to a patient for a routine visit that died the minute I sat down at his bedside. As a hospice nurse, one of my difficult struggles is seeing a patient who is in distress and whom I believe is actively dying, but somehow rallies, gets up and walks to the kitchen and asks what's for dinner. How many times can I give the "he only has a few hours left" speech, without completely throwing the entire family totally off whack?

No human dies the same, death in general is so unpredictable that despite the obvious signs, you cannot be certain that he/she truly only has minutes to live. I've seen enough last breaths to know they are near, but death does not have a time clock, it does not wait for a holiday or a special event to come or to pass… it simply has it's own agenda and happens when it is truly time. And humans, despite how well you may know them, and lovingly want you at their bedside, will wait until that one moment you leave to get a bite to eat to take their last breath. It is not personal, some people just don't want an audience, and some… feel the need to protect you and don't want you to have to see them at that exact moment.

Do I believe they know? Yes. I believe that sometimes, they are completely in control of the exact moment they take their last breath. I also believe that sometimes, they are waiting for one more person to come say goodbye, or for families to come back together, or for fighting to end, or forgiveness to be given.

My mother was a bit of a drama queen. The day she took her last breaths, she had all of her kids gathered around her bed; calling us by our nicknames, saying her farewells… she even called my dad, who happened to be in a hospital bed three cities away, to say goodbye (they had been divorced well over twenty years). She said very dramatically "I am going now", she crossed her arms over her chest and she took her last breaths. There was no struggle, no distress, no lingering apnea or slow drawn out breaths. She just died. And I stood there… totally unprepared for what that might feel like. All of a sudden your mother is no longer here. We were not close, I didn't have that sadness I see so often with others, I wish I did. But I am thankful I did not have to see her struggle.

So I have learned, when I am sitting at the bedside helping a loved one say goodbye, that instead of giving them a time frame, I let them know it's close, it could be soon, and that for right now, they have an opportunity to make it the best last moment they possibly can… and if there happens to be a few more hours, another day… or even longer… those are bonus moments. I think I would regret it more if I didn't say it was close, if I didn't give them that last chance to say a few more words. I am okay with prompting them too early.

It Sucks To Die

I admit it. I get attached. I try so hard not to. This work we do is so intimate and so personal that a deep connection is made relatively quickly. Sometimes it doesn't happen; sometimes they are the patient and I am the nurse, and while I am still compassionate and kind to the end, I don't get that ache when they pass. But sometimes, the connection is made immediately and a bond is built at the first hello. And the ache, the pain I feel when they pass... cuts deep.

I wish I could truly express the feeling I have when I meet a patient for the first time and I look in their eyes and I know they are dying and I know they know they are dying and all I want to do, is to remove their pain and fear and I make an unspoken promise to take their hand and not let it go until their last breath is taken. I give all of me, which can be my worst and best quality. I don't know how to do it any other way. I see their sadness when it's time for me to go and I fill with happy when I see their face light up as I walk in the door. Just knowing they trust me feeds my soul. Some patients I can't wait to see, and leaving after each visit makes me sad; I have a very difficult time leaving at the end of some visits, because I know... this may very well be the last time I see them. I don't think people truly realize how hard this job is, or how personally it effects us or how deeply we give.

I had a patient recently who falls into the category of me becoming too attached. And yes, I became too attached. I walked into her room; she was lying in her bed and looked so weak, and so tired and so frail. It took everything I had not to cry. I cry so easily lately. Not really lately, I just cry easily. Let's be honest... I am emotional and I feel things deeply. Anyway... I was sitting at her bedside and she looked at me and said, "I need you to be brutally honest with me. When am I going to die"? The lump you might be feeling as you read this is exactly the lump I felt when she asked me that. I had about 10 seconds to think about this, wondering what I would want to hear. Dying sucks. People hover around you like a vulture, which feels like they are anticipating your death. You know that they know, but no one says the truths. Everyone tries to be so kind, and thoughtful with their words, but is that the best way to be? I decided to be exactly what she asked of me, and I was brutally honest… "you are going to die, and probably soon… maybe a week, maybe two." And she looked at me and said "thank you". She legitimately thanked me for telling her that she was going to die. How do I process this without completely losing it? But what I took from this is the ways we behave around people who are dying. Without realizing it, we treat them like they are going to die. Could we do this differently? YES!!!! We could stop treating them as though they are fragile, despite the fact that they are. We could create a less dismal environment around them. We can talk TO THEM instead of ABOUT THEM in their presence, and we can ask them directly, and honestly, what they need from us.

Death has become a taboo subject; some people, like myself, talk about it often, while others refuse to talk about it at all, almost avoiding it completely. Even when it reflects something they might be experiencing themselves, they don't let anyone know and feel the need to keep it private. I actually get that, because the thing about death, much like anything else we experience, is that people always have an opinion. But death, especially for the person experiencing it, IS private and personal and intimate and it's a one-time event… I think people deserve the right to have it done the way they are most comfortable with, and if given the chance to voice their wishes, we should respect them.

Imagine if we each took time to tell the people we love, how we would want our death to be. Obviously some things cannot be planned out. We cannot predict our life and certainly not our death. But what if we could ask those we love to not be so heavy, to not whisper at our bedside, but to play certain music, to talk with us instead of about us and most of all… to remind us and those we love about the impact we had on the life we lived. I would want people to talk about the life I lived while at my bedside, to share the stories of the fun we had and the memories we made. I would want to be reminded of the life I lived. And until that time, way before I am on that death bed, I want to live a life, that is filled with memory making; for myself and those I love. I have learned so much about life, while seeing so much death, most importantly is living a life that is fun to talk about and makes people laugh, and smile… and yeah… sometimes cry… but that just means you touched their heart. This life… is a life worth living and I want to be reminded of that before I die.

I had a conversation today with some 20-somethings and we discussed death. Both stated that they didn't want to know what happens when they die, and both admitted that they don't believe in heaven, hell or the afterlife. They just want to live for right now and embrace the right now. BUT… if given a life expectancy of something very short term, they would want the truth. The brutal complete truth. They would want to know they only had a week or two left… because given that time frame, allows them to say the goodbyes, drink the really good whiskey, and die with some dignity and grace.

Dying sucks. Dying without notice, takes our grand finale away from us. But given some notice, given a time frame, allows us the chance to at the very least, do it on our terms. This doesn't take away or remove the pain, the struggle or difficulty of knowing you are about to die. We can't do that. No one can do that. But as humans, could we do a better job at that last goodbye? I believe we can, and I think it starts with being completely truthful.

As a nurse, raise your hand right now if you have been asked to NOT say the word "hospice" around a patient you are about to see? As a hospice nurse, I struggle with this. So basically, you are keeping their death a secret? From them???????????? Is that fair? I don't think so. Why do we do that? Death is not easy on any level, in any mindset, at any age, for any reason. Death cannot be sugar coated, we cannot color it with pretty colors, dress it up in a feather boa and glitter or speak softly in hopes someone doesn't get offended.

Death is the end. It's it. And if given notice… a time frame of sorts… it deserves honesty, respect, kindness and dignity. Death, is final, it deserves a proper farewell if there is the opportunity for that… let's give it bells and whistles, glitter and maybe even a feather boa…. But definitely honesty!

My Mothers Blue Tape Measure

When I was a little girl, my mother used to sew. She was at her sewing machine often. I wish I knew then what I know now about how much that meant to her, or the pleasure she derived from being so creative. I get that now, because I too have found my passion with painting, with writing and even with sewing. I remember always seeing piles of cut fabric, strands of thread and "do-overs" laying on the floor around her and I would think it was just so messy and in my way but what I realize now was how truly beautiful it all was. She used to wear this blue tape measure around her neck like jewelry. I thought she was sloppy... I wish I never thought that. One year, just before school started, she made my brother, my sister and I matching clothes out of the flowered kitchen curtains. I was in the 5th grade and I was so humiliated. We walked to the bus stop in our clothes made of kitchen curtains and I was sure that everyone knew.

When my mother died, we were all going through her things deciding what we wanted to keep. At the time, I wanted nothing. I wasn't close to her, we didn't have a relationship that allowed me to feel sentimental and I regretted that. Death is so darn final. It constantly reminds us of what we didn't do or say at the time we could have. At the moment we were rummaging through her personal belongs was that same moment that I wished I could have changed our relationship, that I too could be feeling some kind of attachment to what she left behind. So I decided to find the things that resonated most with me about her, a few baking tools, some poems she had written and I took the blue measuring tape.

As I grew older and became a mother myself, I too started sewing. I made my kids clothing but not from kitchen curtains. I sat for hours at my sewing machine and while my lines were never straight, I loved creating a new dress for my daughter or MC Hammer pants for my son.

And as they grew up and had their own children, I made quilts for my grand daughters. And yes, the lines are still crooked, but the feelings are still the same. I am proud of what I create and I love the feeling of sitting for hours at the machine, despite the pains in my neck and back. And I think of my mother often.

When I became a nurse, one of the things I need to do at each routine visit, is measure their MAC, which requires a tape measure. So I brought out my mom's old tape measure, which I had never used since she passed away, and I bring it into every patient visit. Each time I pull it out of my bag I get this feeling that almost overwhelms me; I feel like she is right there with me and I smile. Each time, I am reminded of her and the gifts she gave me that at the time I was so unaware of but thankfully, am reminded of now daily. In so many ways, I am so much like her and I just had absolutely no idea.

One day, I was sitting with a patient who was nearing her end. She was able to communicate, but we struggled to find conversation. I pulled out my blue measuring tape and I smiled as I always do and she asked me, "What made you smile like that"? So I shared the story about my mom. This story encouraged her to share about her mom and her childhood. We talked quite a bit that day, and at the next two visits I was able to spend time with her until she passed away. And now, when I go in to see a patient and I pull out the tape measure, I tell them about it. My little blue tape measure, that used to belong to my mom, is a beautiful conversation starter with my patients. I ask them about their own memories and they share with such joy in their faces. Most people want to be reminded to remember. I certainly benefit from it myself. She may not be here with me, but my mom and I are closer now than we ever have been. xo

I Didn't Get To Say Goodbye

I woke up yesterday morning prepared to visit a patient whom I knew was nearing her end. I texted her son and said I was on my way. He texted me back and said she had just passed. My first reaction was to cry because I truly felt a loss; a deep, painful loss from losing someone I had grown to care about. Something happens when you spend time with a person at the end of their lives, and in our case, three times a week for about two months. We talked about our kids, our grandkids, the people we loved, the friends we've lost, and the things that inspired us and brought us joy. We shared open and honest conversation about our personal thoughts about life and death, mostly death.

My second reaction after receiving this news, was this horribly painful feeling of guilt. I didn't get to say goodbye. I had promised her I would be there through her entire process, and all I could think about was that I wasn't there at the end. But I reminded myself about conversations I have had with social workers, chaplains and fellow nurses who have all experienced this feeling. And what we remind one another, is that our goal is to provide beautiful, kind and compassionate care and do whatever we can to ensure that their landing is soft and that those closest to them, feel supported and have the education and resources to be there when they need them the most.

Sometimes we are there at their admission, sometimes a few weeks into their process, sometimes only when they take their last breath. But collectively, in hospice, it is about the team and the work we all do to provide the beautiful care. And I feel certain that as a team we did everything she needed and deserved and I am proud of us for that.

A few days before she passed away, I sat down with her sons and I told them I felt she needed a higher level of care and encouraged them to bring her to our hospice house where she could have around the clock nursing care. With her in agreement, we were able to move her to our hospice house and true to what I had promised, she received the most wonderful care. I need to hold that within and know that while I wasn't there at the end, I did provide her with the very best of care and I am okay with that.

Today I felt a little off, despite my attempt to move through my day with some semblance of grace. I couldn't quite shake the fact that I hadn't yet grieved someone I grew to care about and was truly saddened by her passing. I got into my car, selected my Simon & Garfunkel playlist and made it through The Sound of Silence but when Bridge Over Troubled Water played, I broke down and cried. I reached out to someone I love and confessed my break down. He asked me why. I shared. He responded with "you have a big heart and I hope that never changes". Despite the ache, I hope he's right… I cannot imagine doing the work I do without giving my whole heart, but with that comes ache. So as I learn and grow, I am learning to count on people I love to help me work through my losses and my grief. We cannot do this work alone, whether it is with the support of our team or our family of loved ones, we too need to grieve, to feel and sometimes break down and cry. I know in my heart I did some really good work. I know that we, as a team, did some really good work.

Ask Me How My Day Was

I think one of the most important qualities a person can have, is the ability to truly listen. Have you ever been with someone when you are telling them something that really matters to you, something that is important and valuable and they are on their phone or distracted by something else going on nearby? You know they didn't hear a word you said and certainly don't appreciate the value of the content. It could have been about something trivial like the last movie you just watched, but it could also be about a patient you sat with who touched your heart or tugged at your heartstrings. Regardless of what it is that you have to say, when someone tunes you out, it is hurtful.

I have seen the look on faces as I start to talk about my work and what I do. I understand it is a difficult topic, I understand the fear that surrounds death and it is a taboo subject for many. But when you do this kind of work, when you are at the bedside of someone who takes their very last breath and you hug the loved one of someone who had to say goodbye, for us it isn't about death, it is about life.

Working in hospice on any level, places you in the life of someone who is about to die. This work is personal, it is powerful, it is beautiful and it is hard. And at the end of the day, we need to talk about it. Finding someone to talk to, that doesn't do this kind of work, is not an easy task. I have learned that very rarely does anyone ask me how my day is, because they are afraid I am going to tell them. But I want to tell them, I want to share about the beautifully difficult day I had. I want to share the lessons I learned, or the way it felt to take away the pain or discomfort someone might have experienced. I want to talk about a death that while it could have been really hard, ended up being gentle and kind and I had something to do with their landing being soft. I want to talk about my day. And I really, really want someone to ask me how my day was.

I can't tell you how many dinner tables I have sat at where the conversation went from discussions about food, to movies, to work place gossip and while I sat there listening and even participated, I realize that I didn't have much to offer in the conversation that didn't have something to do with death. I struggle with that, because I feel like maybe I have gotten so immersed in my work I have forgotten how to live a life that doesn't have something to do with death. And while that is probably very close to my reality, my life is not completely wrapped around death. It's way deeper than that. Working around death has opened my eyes to so much more than just death. I have been witness to religions of all kinds; to a faith so strong it kind of blows my mind. I find myself almost envious of people who have such a spiritual commitment. It has encouraged me to ask questions, to read, and to learn. My respect for prayer grows every day. I have also seen love, so much love. And compassion and kindness on levels you can't begin to imagine. Every patient I care for, every family I support and every death I am present for reminds me constantly to embrace life. I see death, but I also see life and I find a deeper appreciate for it every single day.

If you know someone who works in hospice, who is around death, who gives their whole heart to someone else at the most difficult time of their life, I can assure you that they would be very happy you asked about their day. To be present for us, to let us share our day with you, to truly listen to our words is one of the kindest most thoughtful things you could do for us. Xo

Fear Of Dying

Death does not come in a "one size fits all" category; it is not usually predictable, and very rarely planned and it will never become our friend. But the one thing we can all agree on is that most people are afraid of it. Dying is scary. It is that one topic of conversation most people avoid, but in my opinion, probably shouldn't. Talking about death can actually help make it a little less scary.

As a hospice nurse, I am front and center at death often. I have provided care and support for hundreds of patients and their families, doing my best to ensure that their death experience is as gentle and kind as possible. I have seen struggle, I have seen pain, and I have seen the look of anguish come over the face of a loved one who felt helpless and scared. And I have felt peace in my heart when I was able to bring comfort and relief, and did my part to ensure his or her landing was soft. But I do not do this alone. I find myself in awe working with the team of people I do, who make it their goal to relieve pain, discomfort, struggle and fear for every patient in our care.

But who does this for us? I have spent a lot of time thinking about the way someone else might die, but lately I have been questioning my own mortality, spending an unusually large amount of time contemplating my own death and what that might look like. I have imagined it being tragic, which has not been comforting understandably. I think what I am afraid of, is not dying in general, but having a death where I might struggle. And not having a team of hearts around me when it's my time, and not having that kindness and comfort. I am scared…not of dying…but of struggling when I do.

I have also started thinking about what would happen when I die, would my kids know what to do? Would they be able to handle that responsibility? Where would I be buried or would I have my ashes scattered out at sea? What would they do with all of my things? I don't have a lot of money, but I do have some; how can I be sure that my kids get it? So many things to think about and consider; but the one thing I know for sure is that I do not want my kids to have to cut through mountains of red tape to organize my life after I have left it. This leads me to my sudden realization that I need to take care of these things now and I encourage all of you to do the same. It isn't a signature on a death certificate, or a nail in a coffin... so to speak... it is simply a way to not burden your family with all of that paper work and have to make choices on your behalf.

So I started the process and I wrote a letter, which I will make into a legal document, but at least it is a start. I was able to put down on paper what I want and what I don't want. I don't want to be hooked up to machines, I don't want people changing my diapers and I do not want to be fed through a tube. And most of all, I don't want my friends or family to be at my bedside for months just waiting. What I do want is for someone like me to make sure I do not suffer, and for someone like the wonderful people I work with to be there for me and for the people I love.

Just knowing that I wrote it down, that I put it "out there", relieved me of the fear I realized I have had brewing inside of me. Dying doesn't scare me; it is inevitable. We are all going to die. I think my epiphany about being more afraid of struggling at death rather than death itself, really gave me comfort.

I have seen so many family members wait until the last breath has been taken to decide on a funeral home. I have seen family members so afraid of the word "hospice", that they chose not to go that route and instead waited for weeks or months sitting vigil in a hospital room where machines and tubes prolonged a life that was already over.

I hope to live a whole lot longer, and when it is my time, I plan to throw a party to be able to say goodbye personally. I will have all my paperwork in place, in the event I don't get a party or a grand farewell. But one thing I know for sure, I will have a choice of what I want, and what I don't want and it will be done with dignity and kindness. I am not afraid of dying, and now I am less afraid of struggling when I do.

Get your paper work in order; hopefully you get to set it aside for a really long time. More importantly, you are not leaving it up to someone else to figure out for you.

The Guest Of Honor

I went to the funeral of a patient yesterday; this is not something I do often. Once in awhile a patient and their family finds a space inside my heart and when they pass, I experience grief that goes beyond reacting to the experience itself, and truly becomes a personal loss for me, and the ache and sadness is very real.

While I have only attended a few, my experience has been that going to them helps me to find my own closure. That moment you lock eyes with the people left behind, the ones wearing the formal clothing, tissues in hand, receiving hugs from the friends and family who have come from near and far to say their goodbyes, you smile as they mouth "thank you" and while no words have been spoken, you know they are glad you are there.

When we get a new patient, they usually come to us at the very end of their life. Some are in pain, some have lost hair, some cannot speak, some cannot remember and all of them are dying. We don't see them at their best and while we might see a photo or two we really don't know who they once were. At their service, however, we hear about the life they lived, the things they did and the people they loved, who loved them back and will miss them terribly. We are given a quick glimpse of the person before the diagnosis. Sometimes I just sit and listen and smile at the stories shared, and sometimes I cry when they cry, not so much for the loss itself, but for the way the loss has effected the ones left behind.

After the service, I sat down on a bench and watched as this group of people came together to say goodbye. There were a lot of hugs, continued tears and so much laughter, which I know she would have loved. She planned her own party; she asked that people laugh and share stories and that while she might be missed she didn't want it to be sad. Everyone honored her wishes.

An elderly woman came and sat down next to me. She introduced herself as a member of the church and someone who had worked with and will miss the guest of honor. She asked me how I knew her and when I told her I was one of her hospice nurses, she took my hand and said "thank you". She asked how it feels to be there at the end of so many lives, and wanted to know why I do this work; we get asked these questions often. I paused for a moment, I looked around at all the people that loved her and I turned to face this woman and I said, "this work is not easy, and death is not easy, but there is something truly gratifying knowing that this beautiful human, who is struggling more than she ever has before, trusts me to make her last days a little gentler". I do this work, because I believe I was called to.

I said goodbye to the lovely woman who sat down beside me and walked over to my patient's son, who had several people gathered around him, noticing a tear slowly coming down his face. He looked up at me, he left the group and he walked up to me and we hugged. His eyes were filled with tears as he thanked me for the care I provided for his mother but also for him and his brother. He said "we couldn't have done this without you", and I know that isn't true, of course they could have, and it wasn't just me it was our whole team that provided the care, but at that moment I welcomed the words and I appreciated them more than he could ever know. And I said, "it truly was my pleasure, thank you so much for sharing her with us".

As I walked away, I said out loud to myself, "and that is why I do this work". And I smiled.

I've Got Mad Love For Our Volunteers

When you or someone you love receives a Hospice order, it is with the understanding that there is only 6 months or less to live. That alone is a hard pill to swallow, and the process moving forward is so full of the unknown that fear is almost always present. Very rarely is anyone prepared for death and what that might entail.

One of the benefits of having Hospice care, is the team that is assigned and who will collaborate together to make sure fear, pain, and distress is relieved and that you, or your loved one does not feel alone. In some cases, there is a large family presence but it doesn't always happen that way and from my perspective it is those times when our team truly blows me away.

While I have mad love and respect for all members of the team, it is the volunteers who I hold just a tad bit higher than the rest. The way they give so unselfishly to others, fills my heart with happy. I feel honored and blessed to work with our volunteers and know that if they have been to, or are about to see one of my patients, they will be in very good hands. Whether it is sitting completely still, holding a hand, singing or reading to a patient, it is done with such kindness and presence and is a true gift to all of our patients.

I have shared this story before, but it is one worth sharing again. It was Christmas Day and I visited a patient who was actively dying. Alone. He was agitated and restless and his process was anything but peaceful. I stayed for three hours until I felt him calm, but leaving him to die alone was difficult for me. I called our volunteer coordinator and asked if there was any way we could have someone sit with him; and I would have been grateful for just an hour.

A vigil request was sent out to our volunteers and I was pleasantly surprised by how many responded. Volunteers took turns every two hours sitting at his bedside. As he took his very last breath twenty-four hours later, he did it while one volunteer played beautiful music on his hammered dulcimer and another was about to step in for his next shift. They were both fully present for him as he passed away and he did not die alone. My heart is full.

End of life care takes a village; a team of people who each bring a unique and special gift to someone at the end of life and our volunteers play a huge role in this. They are a very important part of the team, usually spending more time with the patient than any of us do and in ways that we are not always able to provide. And while it is usually at the bedside being fully present, it is not always the last hours or days of their life. Often times, our volunteers meet the patient early on when they are still alert and oriented and just need someone to talk to, someone who will listen, to be a friend and a companion.

I remember a patient who looked forward to every Wednesday when her volunteer brought ice cream, another who enjoyed visits from his volunteer who brought his dog, and so many family members who appreciated the visits because it meant their loved one was safe and cared for and they could step away and run an errand or just take a few minutes to breathe. Everyone benefits from the volunteers who visit, the patient, the family, and the team.

The peace, the comfort, and the gentle kindness our volunteers bring, is so important to the work we do and a day does not go by that I do not feel honored to share space with them. I admire them, I respect them and from the very depths of my heart I say "thank you" to them.

What Do You Want To Do Before You Die?

I was having a conversation with a patient the other day about the things she wished she had done before she got sick. She talked about the places she wished she had traveled to, and the things she wished she had done. When her granddaughter was about 5, they used to play a game where she would bring out an old globe, spin it around and let her granddaughter pick a place for it to stop. They would create this imaginary adventure to whatever country it landed on and spend hours talking about what they ate, what they wore, who they met and what trouble they would get in together. She started to cry as she was sharing this story, and she said, "we never went anywhere together. I never traveled anywhere. I wish I had done more about what I talked about doing".

I think we all have our own version of a bucket list; things we want to do in this lifetime. But most of us don't see a deadline of time that these things have to be accomplished, and we tend to put them off until later. A few years ago I decided to act on my bucket list. Perhaps it was enhanced by the job I do and how fragile I perceive life, but however it was brought on, I benefitted from it. I bravely booked a trip to Spain and walked two hundred and ten miles of the Camino on my own. I talked, I laughed, and I cried with complete strangers, and I came back a better version of myself. It was the most amazing adventure of my life. The next year I went to Peru for a few weeks with my son and daughter; we took airplanes, busses, boats, and trains and we traveled through city after city learning about Peru and the amazing gifts it had to offer. One of my personal take-a-ways was the way they celebrate life so fully. Again I came home a wiser, more enlightened person.

Then I hurt my shoulder and was unable to travel, and I felt a sense of loss because I couldn't go anywhere. This made me think about my bucket list, things I want to do before I die and I realized it wasn't just about traveling… my thoughts took me to things I don't want to leave behind when I die… such as regrets, words unspoken, etc.

I took a class awhile back, taught by Shaman Linda Fitch; our first assignment was to write our Eulogy. Have you ever done that? Have you ever thought about what people would say about you when you are gone? I wrote my Eulogy that night and it occurred to me that I was not quite living a life that would make a really great Eulogy. I think I am kind, mostly honest, and I do good work in my world… but it's more than that. It's about the message I want to leave behind, the lessons for my kids and my grandkids. I want to make a difference, be a positive change and leave behind something big.

While there are things I could have done differently in my past, I have chosen not to dwell on that. Everything I have done, good or bad, has led me exactly where I am now and I really like where I am now. So I have no regrets. There are no do-overs in life, and we shouldn't put our wishes in a bucket and hope some day we fulfill them… instead I think we should live a full, good life right now. Make memories right now. Say and do the good, kind, wonderful things RGHT NOW. And yes, take trips and see and do amazing things…. But do them now.

What do I want to do before I die? I want to live a really full life. I want to see my kids live a full and beautiful life. I want to watch my grandkids grow up and blow my mind. I want to make moments matter, reassure my family and friends how much I love them, and I want to learn and grow and continue to evolve every single day. I want to make a difference, I want to encourage change and inspire those around me to do the same. I want to live THIS life, which is MY life, right now.

Don't wish things were different. Don't wish you could do or say things. Wishing doesn't make them happen, YOU make them happen. Get out there and do it... this is it, at least in this mindset. This is your life...live it, enjoy it, embrace it. Make some really awesome memories!!! Don't waste a second. Live your life right now!!!

Life After Death

After someone takes their last breath, I stay with the family and I provide comfort, support and active listening. I have a number of tasks I handle for them. I usually make the call to the funeral home, if they've made that arrangement, or assist them if they haven't. You would be surprised how many people do not make that arrangement ahead of time. I tell them how to dispose of the medications, both opened and unused. Which by the way, if you have never experienced this, is one the largest wastes I have ever seen; so much medication is disposed of, some that has never even been opened. I encourage them to welcome the support of our bereavement counselors even if it is months after. And I always offer to bathe them; sometimes the family says "no", sometimes they will participate and sometimes I do it alone. Bathing is a very important ritual for me; there is something truly beautiful about gently bathing someone after they have passed.

As I gather my things and prepare to leave, it feels like time stands still as I say goodbye to those left behind. Whether I have known the patient, their family and/or friends for weeks, days, or just a few hours, the moments before, during and after a death are some of the most powerful and emotional moments for me. They are intimate, delicate, and sensitive. As I have written so many times before, telling someone the last breath has been taken and acknowledging this person has passed, is one of the hardest parts of my job. It is no secret this human is about to die but regardless of how prepared everyone is, those words resonate hard; it feels as though their entire world has come crashing down on them. As if they had absolutely no idea this was about to happen, and I am the one giving the bad news.

But because we shared something so intimate, the moment passes quickly from me being the bearer of bad news, to the reminder of me being the one that held their hand through the most difficult moment of their life. I usually try to hold back my tears, saving them for later when I am alone and no one can see. But sometimes I cry with them, because while I was not personally involved with them up until this moment, their emotions always elicit a response within.

The moment they walk me to the door is also hard because they don't usually want me to leave. It sometimes feels like they are afraid to be alone, to move forward without the support. I held their hands, I guided them through every step and I helped remove their fear. They knew that as soon I walked out that door, they would need to do the rest on their own, and sometimes, at least early on, it is really, really hard to do. I sometimes call them a day or two later, to check in. They are much stronger by then, and for the most part doing okay. They are thankful and express gratitude, which always fills my heart. Our bereavement team follows up with them as well, even when they say they won't need it, most times, they welcome it with very open arms.

What I have noticed is that it is usually many days, or weeks, and sometimes, months after when they have the real struggle. They've been busy with funeral arrangements and legal stuff, family gatherings, and cleaning out everything that had anything to do with them while they were alive. That is busy work that while difficult and emotional, can also be a much-needed distraction while they navigate the loss. It has been my experience that it is after this time, when emotions come back up and in many ways are even more painful. It feels like everyone expects you to be fine and "over it" so you keep things to yourself. But the truth is, at least from what I have seen, once all the busy distractions are over and you find yourself alone with your thoughts, all you can do is think. And that is when they need us the most.

When someone loses someone they love, the pain doesn't go away with time; sometimes it might calm for a bit but it comes back when they least expect it. Don't assume they are fine even if they say they are. Keep checking in. Let them know you are there. They might not want to talk about it, but I can almost guarantee they would really love to know that they haven't been forgotten. Because what usually happens, is that everyone is there in the beginning, but one by one, as time fades… so do the people in your corner.

The thing about losing someone you love is that the pain and ache doesn't ever really go away. You don't just stop thinking about them. Some days are better than others, and some days are worse. And while life goes on and time passes by, we hope that the one that is hurting the most starts to feel a little better, but it is usually only temporary, because the thing about grief is that it doesn't have an expiration date. Our job, as their friend or family member, is to keep checking in; on the holidays, the birthdays, the anniversary of each year after they've passed and sometimes "just because".

There is life after death for those that have been left behind but life will never be the same for them. Healing takes time, and it is a process that does not come with a guidebook. No one actually gets over it, and no one forgets, please don't expect them to. Love them, support them and be patient with them.

Thank you very much for taking the time to read my book.

If I can give any advice to you, it would be to allow everyone you love to have a choice; their own, individual, independent choice. This can be how they live, how they love, and yes, even how the die. None of us have the right to push our thoughts and opinions onto someone else and I think the less we do that, the more comfortable people will be about sharing what it is they want or need.

I believe our role is to create a safe place for the people we love to share their thoughts and needs with us, whether or not it is something we might support or believe in. To be a safe place for someone is a gift, a priceless, wonderful gift.

Death is hard enough, but feeling forced to do it the way someone else feels is right, is not fair or kind. I understand we all have our own opinions but they are not always going to be something someone else feels and we should not take it upon ourselves to push them on to someone else. I have seen so many people in their last days, afraid to be honest about what they want or don't want, for fear of disappointing someone they love. And while that is kind and thoughtful on their part, they end up struggling emotionally and sometimes physically because of it.

If someone you love has been given a terminal diagnosis, ask them what they want and what they might need from you and if they tell you they want to do something you do not agree with, just tell them you love them and you will be there for them any way that you can. And before this happens, before you or someone you love is told their time is short, live the fullest, most wonderful life you possibly can. Love yourself and one another fiercely. Be kind. Be compassionate. Be thankful, and grateful. And make lots and lots of wonderful memories…

With so much gratitude, Gabby

Made in the USA
Monee, IL
05 May 2024